Workbook to Accompany

The Medical Manager®

STUDENT EDITION

VERSION 10.31

D0218816

Workbook to Accompany

The Medical Manager®

STUDENT EDITION
VERSION 10.31

Maria Stio, *Professor*
Briarcliffe College, New York

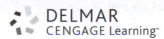
DELMAR
CENGAGE Learning™

Australia • Brazil • Japan • Korea • Mexico • Singapore • Spain • United Kingdom • United states

DELMAR
CENGAGE Learning™

Workbook to Accompany The Medical Manager® Student Edition Version 10.31
Maria Stio

Vice President, Career and Professional Editorial: Dave Garza

Director of Learning Solutions: Matthew Kane

Senior Acquisitions Editor: Rhonda Dearborn

Managing Editor: Marah Bellegarde

Product Manager: Jadin Babin-Kavanaugh

Editorial Assistant: Chiara Astriab

Vice President, Career and Professional Marketing: Jennifer McAvey

Executive Marketing Manager: Wendy Mapstone

Senior Marketing Manager: Nancy Bradshaw

Marketing Coordinator: Erica Ropitzky

Production Director: Carolyn Miller

Production Manager: Andrew Crouth

Content Project Manager: Thomas Hefferman

Senior Art Director: Jack Pendelton

For more information, contact Delmar Learning, 5 Maxwell Drive, Clifton Park, NY 12065
Or find us on the World Wide Web at http://www.delmarlearning.com

For permission to use material from this text or product, contact us by
Tel (800) 730-2214
Fax (800) 730-2215
www.delmar.cengage.com

ISBN-13: 978-1-4283-3613-1
ISBN-10: 1-4283-3613-3

NOTICE TO THE READER

Printed in the United States of America
5 6 7 8 9 10 11 16 15 14 13 12

CONTENTS

P R E F A C E

INTRODUCTION

This is a workbook designed to provide additional practice for The Medical Manager Student Edition, Version 10.31. The purpose for this workbook is to supply the student with additional exercises that build on the tasks and skills taught in each unit of the Student Edition. By completing these additional exercises, the student can reinforce skills learned and gain confidence by demonstrating the ability to use The Medical Manager software.

DEVELOPMENT OF TEXT

This workbook was developed to provide students with supplementary material to complement the course-work from The Medical Manager Student Edition, Version 10.31. Many times a student needs additional assignments in order to understand a concept or practice a skill. Other times, a student may want to work on additional assignments in order to gain more experience and knowledge. The idea behind this workbook was to assist all students so that they may become proficient in using The Medical Manager. In addition, the instructor may use this workbook for competency exercises, unit tests, or to evaluate a student's progress.

ORGANIZATION

Each unit in the Student Edition focuses on specific tasks. The workbook exercises relate back to the skills covered in each unit, providing situations that help to emphasize key points and highlight certain features.

The workbook exercises are designed with a brief explanation of the tasks expected to be completed, specific exercise goals, and relevant questions to consider before entering data. Comprehensive exercises can be found in Unit 10 to help the student feel self-assured as well as allow the instructor to evaluate a student's understanding of The Medical Manager.

FEATURES

All exercises are clearly identified in the Contents for easy access. If a student is struggling with a particular task or wants to complete additional work, the Contents can be used to locate exercises utilizing the designed function.

In addition to the exercises, images of The Medical Manager screens are provided in order to check data entered. By using the screen images, a student can identify any errors in entry and/or ensure the accuracy of each posting.

HOW TO USE

A student can easily use this workbook to enhance the skills learned from the Student Edition. For best benefits, after completing all units from The Medical Manager Student Edition, Version 10.31, it is suggested that students follow through all the unit exercises provided in the workbook. In this way, a student will gain optimal experience at using this software.

IMPORTANT NOTE FOR INSTRUCTORS

Please note that because of the real-world limitations on advancing the date in Version 10.31 of The Medical Manager software, the workbook exercises must be started *after* the core text exercises have been fully completed. For more information, please see the instructor's manual for more details.

Instructors may choose to use this workbook for unit tests. Each exercise is given a brief explanation or goal of the task at hand; however, step-by-step instructions are not provided. In this way, a student will need to retain and recall information provided from the Student Edition exercises.

Whatever the needs of the individual student or entire class, The Medical Manager Student Edition Workbook provides the tools necessary to be a successful user of The Medical Manager software program.

ABOUT THE AUTHOR

Maria Stio is a professor at Briarcliffe College, New York. Prior to teaching, she had worked in pediatrics for nine years as a medical receptionist, medical biller, and medical assistant. Later she worked at a clinic as an office manager; as well as provided training at various sites on The Medical Manager software. She has grown with The Medical Manager from the DOS version to version 10.31.

Maria Stio has been an educator for the past thirteeen years, with a specialty in the medical field. Among various computer courses, she teaches medical terminology, medical transcription, medical coding and insurance procedures, and The Medical Manager software program to students preparing to enter the medical office profession.

UNIT 1

Using The Medical Manager

EXERCISE 1: FLOW OF INFORMATION IN A MEDICAL OFFICE

Answer the following questions based on your understanding and review of Unit 1.

1. Discuss the importance of the flow of information in a medical office.

_____

_____

_____

_____

_____

2. Define overbooking and describe why it is not recommended.

_____

_____

_____

_____

_____

3. Name three situations that you would consider an emergency for a patient.

1. _____

2. _____

3. _____

4. What information is found on an encounter form?

_____

_____

5. Describe the main goal of managed care plans.

_____

_____

_____

6. What does "PCP" stand for?

_____

7. Name five tasks that can be completed using The Medical Manager software.

    1. _____

    2. _____

    3. _____

    4. _____

    5. _____

8. Describe the advantages of using the direct chaining feature.

_____

_____

_____

_____

9. What edit key will erase all characters in the field?

_____

10. What key is used to process data and save your work?

_____

11. Discuss the importance of the File Maintenance menu.

_____

_____

_____

_____

12. What key is the same as keying a "?" to open help windows?

_____

13. What type of medical codes are CPT-4 and ICD-9?

_____

14. What is the preferred method for exiting The Medical Manager Student Edition?

_____

_____

_____

15. What does a fatal error indicate?

_____

_____

_____

U N I T 2

Building Your
Patient File

In the unit exercises that follow (Accounts 300–304), you will be entering new patient accounts from the patient registration forms provided.

EXERCISE 1: PATIENT WITH GUARANTOR INSURANCE

THERESA WALTERS; ACCOUNT 300

1. Before attempting data entry, study the patient registration form in Figure 2-1. Answer the following questions.

   a. Who is the guarantor for the account? _____

   b. What is the relationship between the guarantor and the patient? _____

   c. Is Extended Information provided for Theresa Walters? _____

   d. How many insurance policies are there for the account? _____

   e. Who is the policyholder of the insurance? _____

Figure 2-1   Patient Registration – Theresa Walters

Patient Registration Form

Sydney Carrington & Associates
34 Sycamore Street ● Madison, CA 95653

FOR OFFICE USE ONLY	
ACCOUNT NO.:	300
DOCTOR:	#1
BILL TYPE:	11
EXTENDED INFO.:	2

TODAY'S DATE: _06/02/2008_

PATIENT INFORMATION

Walters	_Theresa_	_L._	
PATIENT LAST NAME	FIRST NAME	MI	SUFFIX

EMPLOYER OR SCHOOL NAME

MAILING ADDRESS   CITY   STATE   ZIP CODE

EMPLOYER OR SCHOOL ADDRESS   CITY   STATE   ZIP CODE

_F_	_05/10/1974_	_Married_	_132-17-0427_
SEX (M/F)	DATE OF BIRTH	MARITAL STATUS	SOC. SEC. #

EMPLOYER OR SCHOOL PHONE NUMBER

Wife

HOME PHONE   RELATIONSHIP TO GUARANTOR

Katrina Johnson, M.D.

REFERRED BY

GUARANTOR INFORMATION

Walters	_Charles_	_—_	_M_	_03/19/1970_	_Married_	_145-98-0424_
RESPONSIBLE PARTY LAST NAME	FIRST NAME	MI	SEX (M/F)	DATE OF BIRTH MARITAL STATUS		SOC. SEC. #

3 Jefferson Avenue		_Otis Electronics_
MAILING ADDRESS	STREET ADDRESS (IF DIFFERENT)	EMPLOYER NAME

Floral City	_CA_	_94064_	_18 Saxon Avenue_
CITY	STATE	ZIP CODE	EMPLOYER ADDRESS

_(916) 752-9612_	_(917) 529-7788_	_Madison_	_CA_	_95653_
(AREA CODE) HOME PHONE	(AREA CODE) WORK PHONE	CITY	STATE	ZIP CODE

PRIMARY INSURANCE

Cross and Shield Ins.	_Same_
NAME OF PRIMARY INSURANCE COMPANY	ADDRESS (IF DIFFERENT)

435 Embarcadero	_Same_		
ADDRESS	CITY	STATE	ZIP CODE

Madison	_CA_	_95653_	_(800) 345-7689_	_145-98-0424_
CITY	STATE	ZIP CODE	PRIMARY INSURANCE PHONE NUMBER	SOC. SEC. #

_7354119_	_Otis_	_Self_
IDENTIFICATION #	GROUP NAME AND/OR #	WHAT IS THE RESPONSIBLE PARTY'S RELATIONSHIP TO THE INSURED?

Charles Walters

INSURED PERSON'S NAME (IF DIFFERENT FROM THE RESPONSIBLE PARTY)

SECONDARY INSURANCE

NAME OF SECONDARY INSURANCE COMPANY   ADDRESS (IF DIFFERENT)

ADDRESS   CITY   STATE   ZIP CODE

CITY   STATE   ZIP CODE   SECONDARY INSURANCE PHONE NUMBER   SOC. SEC. #

IDENTIFICATION #   GROUP NAME AND/OR #   WHAT IS THE RESPONSIBLE PARTY'S RELATIONSHIP TO THE INSURED?

INSURED PERSON'S NAME (IF DIFFERENT FROM THE RESPONSIBLE PARTY)

I hereby consent for Sydney Carrington & Associates, P.A. to use or disclose my health information to carry out treatment, payment, and health care operations. I authorize the use of this signature on all insurance submissions. I understand that I am financially responsible for all charges whether or not paid by the insurance. I acknowledge receipt of the practice's privacy policy.

Theresa L. Walters	_06/02/2008_
PATIENT SIGNATURE	DATE

2. Based on the information found on the patient registration form, add Theresa Walters as a new patient. Compare your screens to Figures 2-2 through 2-6.

Figure 2-2 Guarantor Information

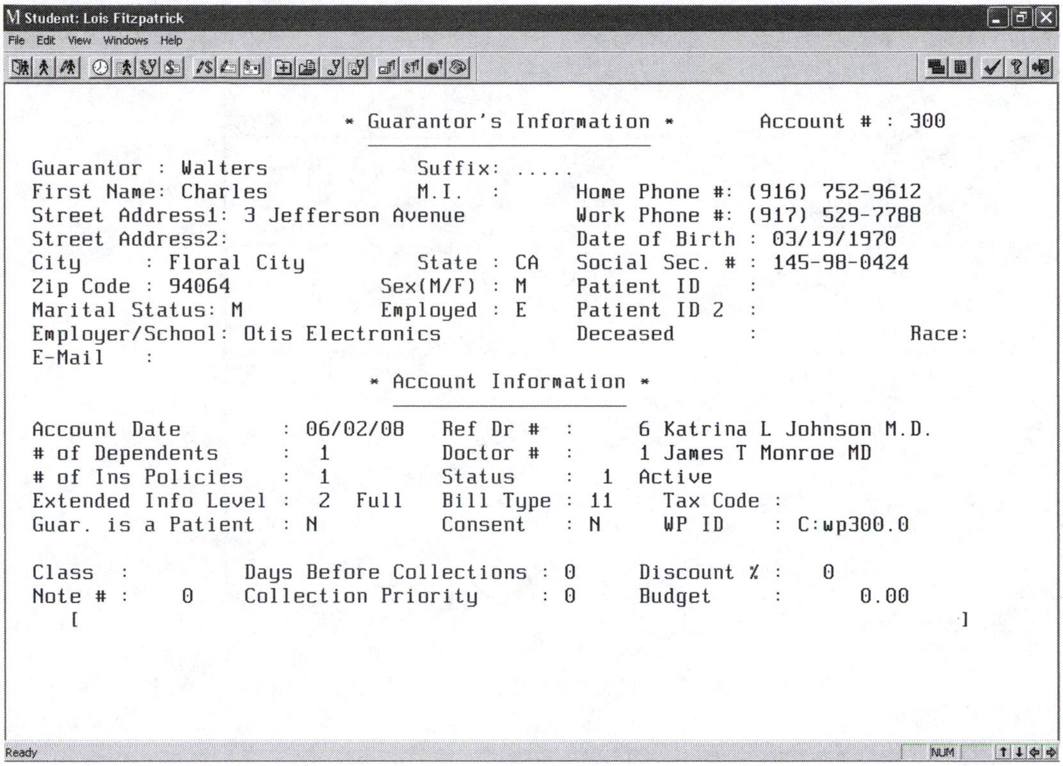

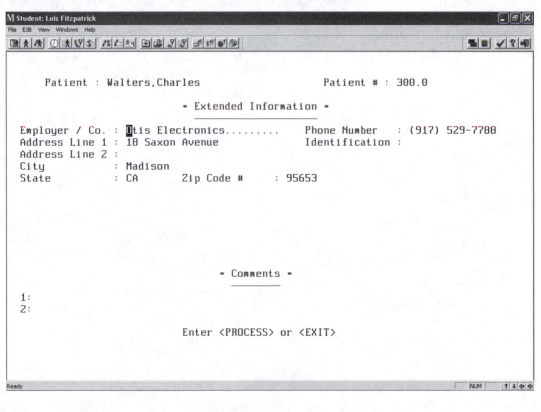

Figure 2-3 Guarantor Extended Information

Figure 2-4   Theresa Walters Information

```
M Student: Lois Fitzpatrick                                        _ 🗗 X
File  Edit  View  Windows  Help
🔲🚶🏃⏲🔧💲 /S📑🔲 ⊞📄♩♫ ⊿♬●♻             ■▦ ✓?📤

   Account #: 300              Dependent Information           [Walters]


        Dependent #                : 1
        Dependent Last Name        : Walters          Suffix : .....
        Dependent First Name       : Theresa          M.I. : L
        Dependent Date of Birth    : 05/10/1974
        Dependent Sex (M/F)        : F
        Relation to Guarantor      : W
        Social Security Number     : 132-17-0427
        Patient ID                 :
        Patient ID 2               :
        Default Doctor #           :    1 James T Monroe MD
        Referring Doctor #         :    6 Katrina L Johnson M.D.
        Extended Information Level :  0  None
        WP File ID                 : C:wp300.1
        Marital Status             : M
        Race                       :
        Employment/Student Status  :              Consent  : Y
        Date Became a Patient      : 06/02/2008    Deceased :
        E-Mail :



Ready                                                    NUM   ↑↓↩➡
```

Figure 2-5   Insurance Policy – Walters

```
M Student: Lois Fitzpatrick                                        _ 🗗 X
File  Edit  View  Windows  Help
🔲🚶🏃⏲🔧💲 /S📑🔲 ⊞📄♩♫ ⊿♬●♻             ■▦ ✓?📤

   Account #: 300      Insurance Policy Information for 1 of 1   [Walters,Charles]


 Policyholder  : 0.    [Walters, Charles      ]
 Carrier Code  : CASA    [Cross and Shield Plans   ]
 Plan #        : 6       Plan Code:          Form #  : 1   Fmt # : 1
 Plan Name     : Cross and Shield Ins Plan   EMC ID 1 : 8499E89S489489
 Attention     :                             EMC ID 2 :
 Street Address: 435 Embarcadero             Deductible:   500.00
 City,State,Zip: Madison       CA   95653    Program  : BL BC/BS
 Phone #       : (800) 345-7689   Class : EMC  Assignment - Dr : Y  Pat : Y
 Group Number  :                             Ins ID # : 7354119
 Group Name    : Otis                        User Note :
 Policy Dates - From :        To :           Copay Ext :     Ins Type: GP
      Insured Party #       : 0              Rpt Group :
      Last Name or Company  : Walters               Suffix:
      First Name, M.I.      : Charles         Sex  : M  DOB : 03/19/1970
      Address               : 3 Jefferson Avenue
      City,St,Zip           : Floral City   CA   94064
      Insured Party ID #    : 145-98-0424      Phone : (916) 752-9612
      Insured's Employer    : Otis Electronics
      Employer Ins Plan     : Y

      Enter Dependent # of Policyholder, 0 for Guarantor, or '?' for Help


Ready                                                    NUM   ↑↓↩➡
```

Figure 2-6 Insurance Coverage – Walters

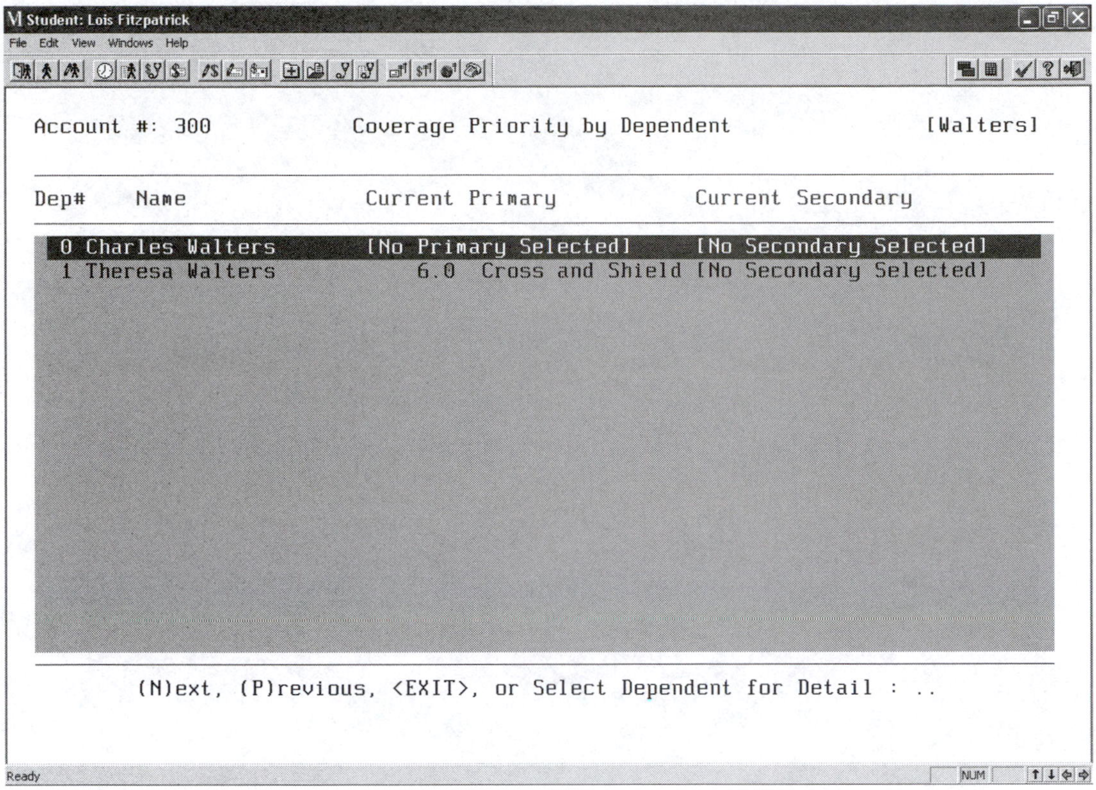

EXERCISE 2: PATIENT WITH DIFFERENT LAST NAME AND DIFFERENT INSURED PARTY

HELENA CARLOS; ACCOUNT 301

1. Before attempting data entry, study the patient registration form in Figure 2-7. Answer the following questions.

    a. What is the relationship between the guarantor, patient, and policyholder? _____

    b. In the Employed field, will Helena be (E)mployed, (P)art Time Student, or (F)ull Time Student? _____

    c. What is the address of the policyholder? _____

    Is it different from the guarantor's address? _____

Figure 2-7 Patient Registration – Helena Carlos

2. Based on the information found on the patient registration form, add Helena Carlos as a new patient. Compare your screens to Figures 2-8 through 2-12.

Figure 2-8 Guarantor Information – Rojas

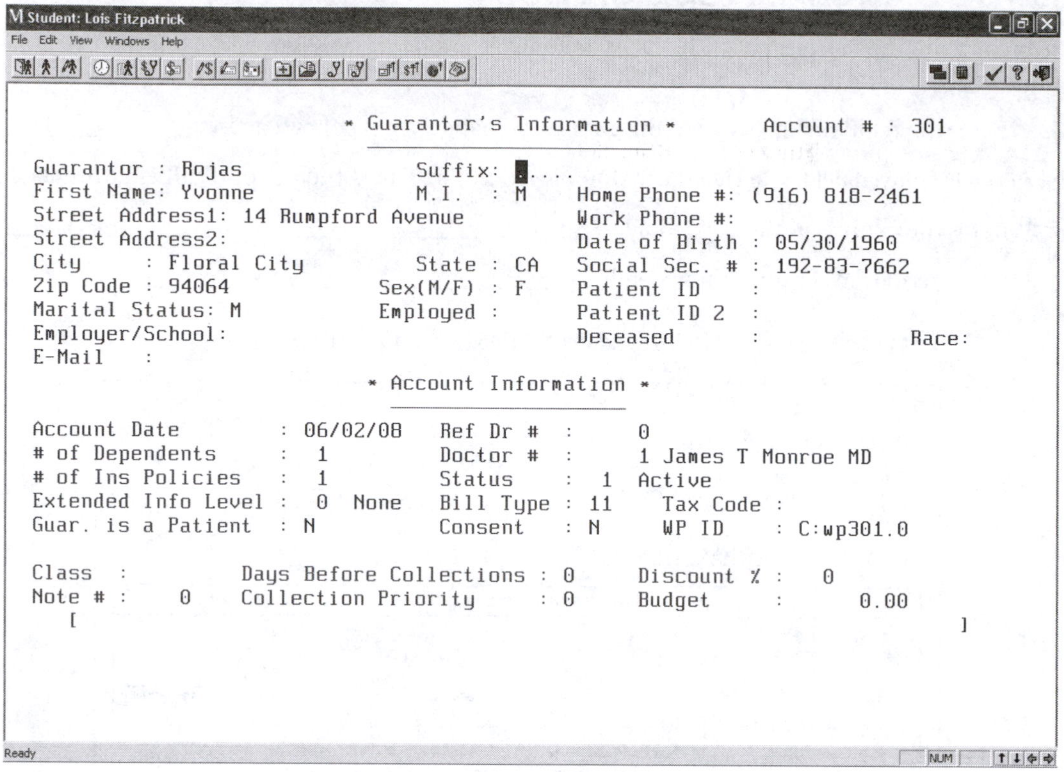

Figure 2-9 Dependent Information – Carlos

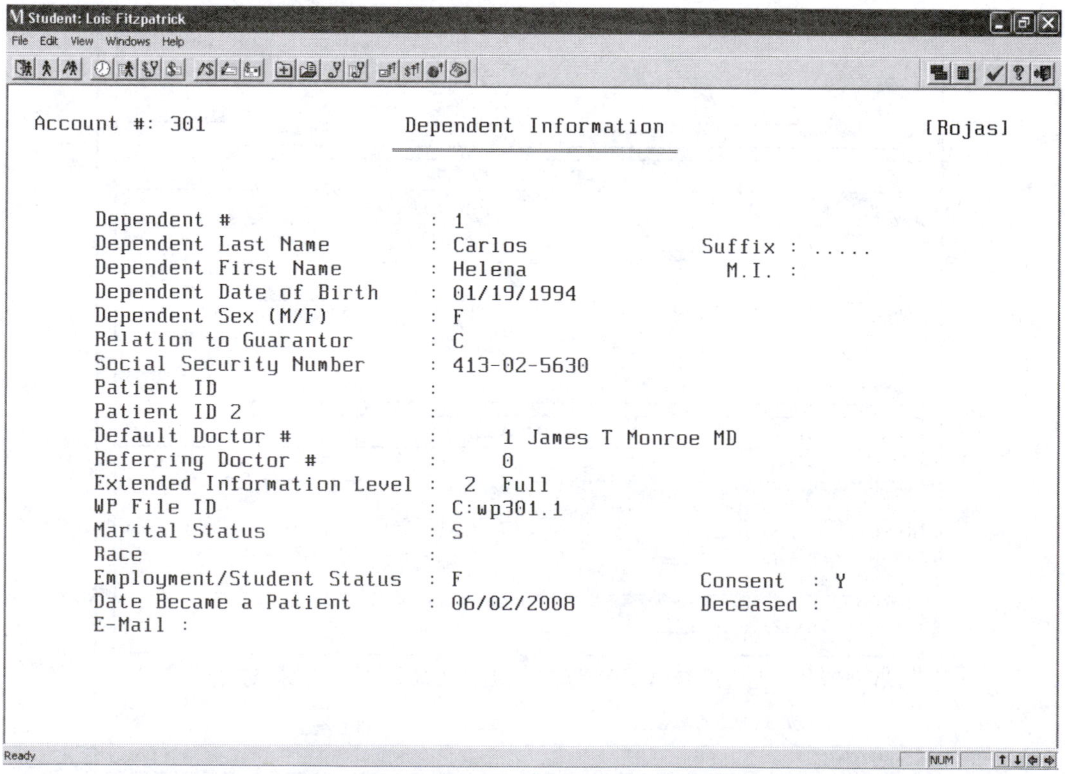

Figure 2-10 Extended Information – Carlos

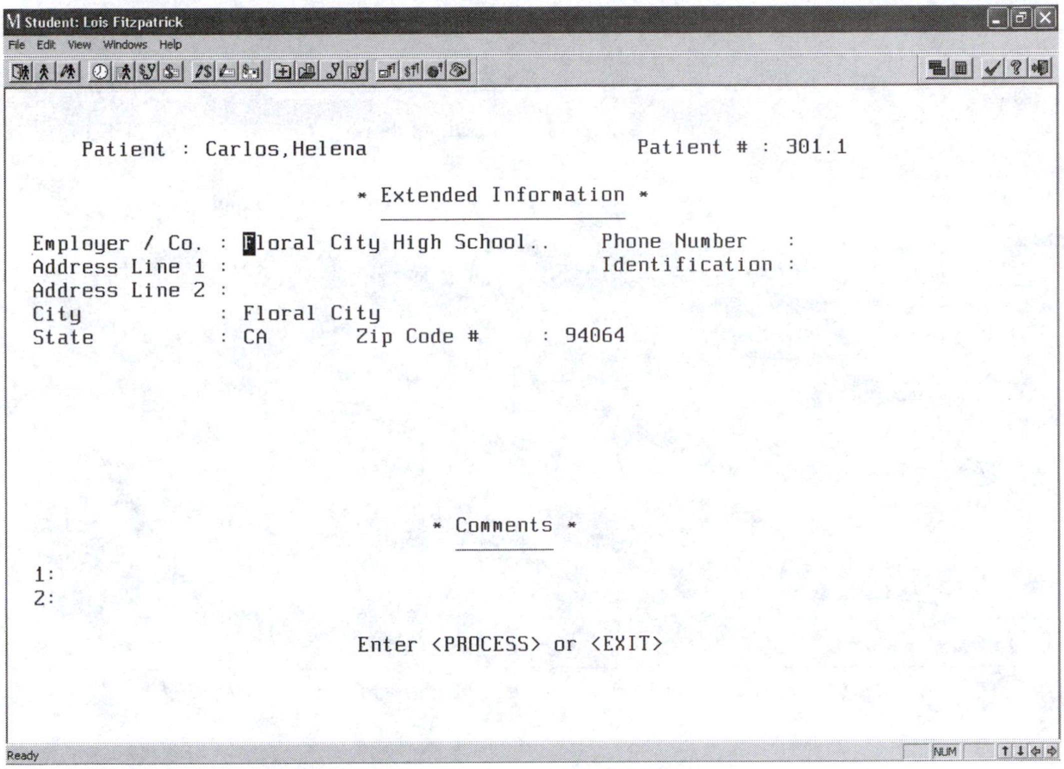

```
M Student: Lois Fitzpatrick                                          _  □  X
File  Edit  View  Windows  Help

        Patient : Carlos,Helena                 Patient # : 301.1

                       * Extended Information *
                       _____

   Employer / Co. : Floral City High School..   Phone Number   :
   Address Line 1 :                             Identification :
   Address Line 2 :
   City           : Floral City
   State          : CA        Zip Code #    : 94064




                              * Comments *
                              _____

   1:
   2:

                     Enter <PROCESS> or <EXIT>



Ready                                                    NUM    ↑ ↓ ⇔ ⇨
```

NOTE: _Insured party numbers are assigned by the computer and may differ from the number shown in Figure 2-11._

Figure 2-11 Insurance Policy Information – Carlos

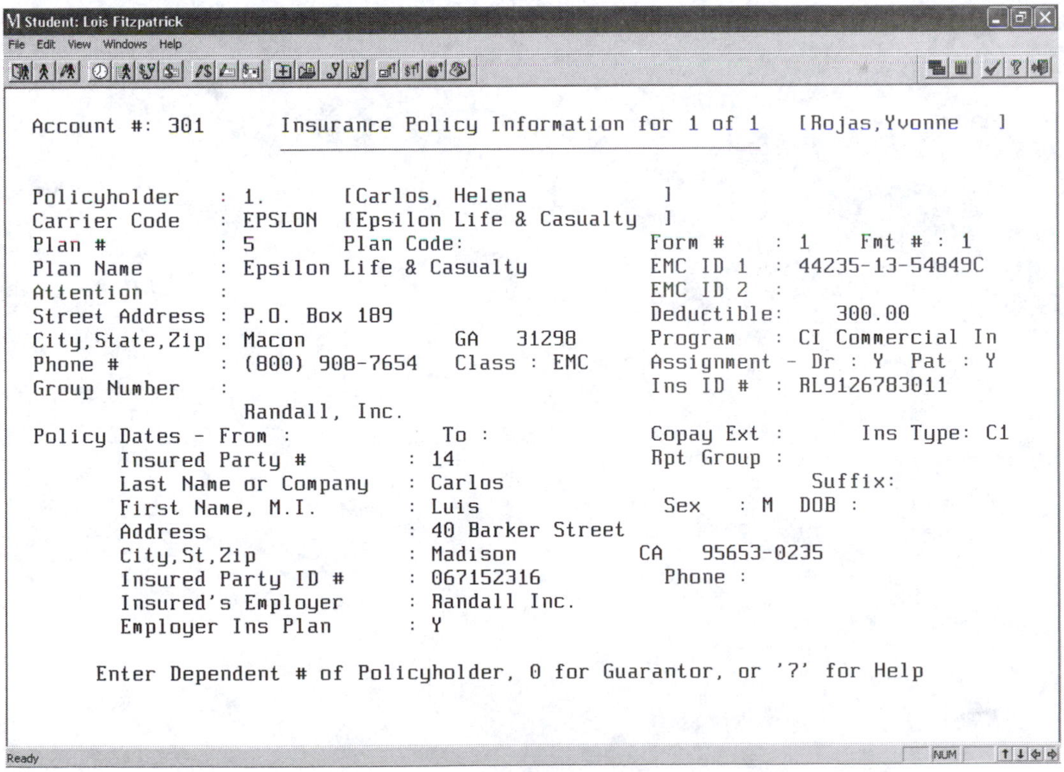

```
M Student: Lois Fitzpatrick                                          _  □  X
File  Edit  View  Windows  Help

  Account #: 301      Insurance Policy Information for 1 of 1   [Rojas,Yvonne  ]


   Policyholder   : 1.      [Carlos, Helena        ]
   Carrier Code   : EPSLON  [Epsilon Life & Casualty ]
   Plan #         : 5       Plan Code:          Form #    : 1   Fmt # : 1
   Plan Name      : Epsilon Life & Casualty     EMC ID 1 : 44235-13-54849C
   Attention      :                             EMC ID 2 :
   Street Address : P.O. Box 189                Deductible:    300.00
   City,State,Zip : Macon        GA   31298      Program    : CI Commercial In
   Phone #        : (800) 908-7654  Class : EMC  Assignment - Dr : Y  Pat : Y
   Group Number   :                              Ins ID #   : RL9126783011
                    Randall, Inc.
   Policy Dates - From :         To :           Copay Ext :      Ins Type: C1
       Insured Party #       : 14               Rpt Group :
       Last Name or Company  : Carlos                         Suffix:
       First Name, M.I.      : Luis             Sex  : M  DOB :
       Address               : 40 Barker Street
       City,St,Zip           : Madison          CA   95653-0235
       Insured Party ID #    : 067152316         Phone :
       Insured's Employer    : Randall Inc.
       Employer Ins Plan     : Y

         Enter Dependent # of Policyholder, 0 for Guarantor, or '?' for Help


Ready                                                    NUM    ↑ ↓ ⇔ ⇨
```

Figure 2-12 Insurance Coverage – Carlos

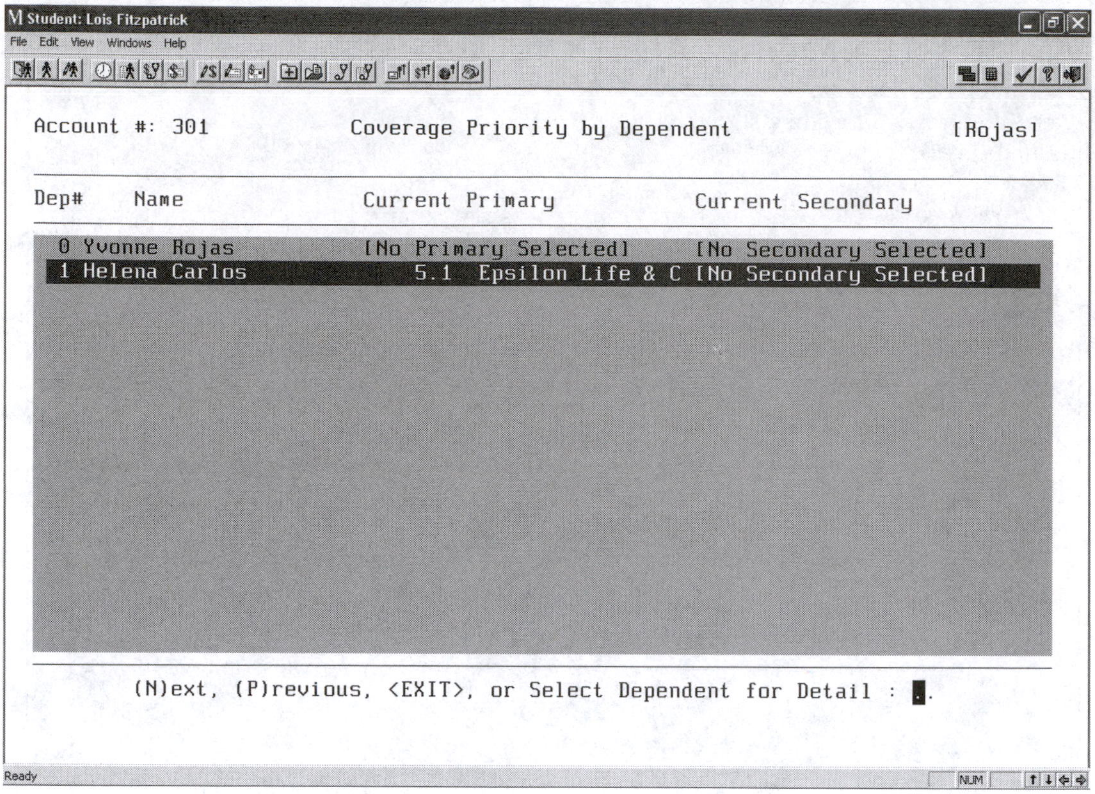

EXERCISE 3: GUARANTOR IS PATIENT

EDWARD GLENMORE; ACCOUNT 302

1. Before attempting data entry, study the patient registration form in Figure 2-13. Answer the following questions.
   a. What is the address of the patient? ______________________
   What will appear on Address Line 1? ______________________
   What will appear on Address Line 2? ______________________
   b. Who is the policyholder of the insurance? ______________________

Figure 2-13 Patient Registration – Edward Glenmore

Patient Registration Form

Sydney Carrington & Associates
34 Sycamore Street • Madison, CA 95653

TODAY'S DATE: 06/02/2008

FOR OFFICE USE ONLY	
ACCOUNT NO.:	302
DOCTOR:	#2
BILL TYPE:	11
EXTENDED INFO.:	2

PATIENT INFORMATION

PATIENT LAST NAME: Glenmore | FIRST NAME: Edward | MI: R. | SUFFIX:
MAILING ADDRESS: | CITY: | STATE: | ZIP CODE:
SEX (M/F): M | DATE OF BIRTH: 08/16/1950 | MARITAL STATUS: Married | SOC. SEC. #: 147-53-1990
HOME PHONE: | RELATIONSHIP TO GUARANTOR: Self
EMPLOYER OR SCHOOL NAME: Powers Lighting, Inc.
EMPLOYER OR SCHOOL ADDRESS: P.O. Box 426 | CITY: Madison | STATE: CA | ZIP CODE: 95653-0235
EMPLOYER OR SCHOOL PHONE NUMBER: (916) 334-9800
REFERRED BY:

GUARANTOR INFORMATION

RESPONSIBLE PARTY LAST NAME: Glenmore | FIRST NAME: Edward | MI: R. | SEX (M/F): M
MAILING ADDRESS: P.O. Box 1624 | STREET ADDRESS (IF DIFFERENT): 12 Kenway Street
CITY: Madison | STATE: CA | ZIP CODE: 95653-0235
(AREA CODE) HOME PHONE: (916) 707-1531 | (AREA CODE) WORK PHONE: (916) 334-9800
DATE OF BIRTH: 08/16/1950 | MARITAL STATUS: Married | SOC. SEC. #: 147-53-1990
EMPLOYER NAME: Powers Lighting, Inc.
EMPLOYER ADDRESS: P.O. Box 426
CITY: Madison | STATE: CA | ZIP CODE: 95653-0235

PRIMARY INSURANCE

NAME OF PRIMARY INSURANCE COMPANY: Fringe Benefits Center
ADDRESS: 123 Mission Corners
CITY: San Mates | STATE: TX | ZIP CODE: 78723
IDENTIFICATION #: 14876PL | GROUP NAME AND/OR #: Powers
INSURED PERSON'S NAME (IF DIFFERENT FROM THE RESPONSIBLE PARTY): Powers Lighting, Inc.
ADDRESS (IF DIFFERENT): P.O. Box 426
CITY: Madison | STATE: CA | ZIP CODE: 95653-0235
PRIMARY INSURANCE PHONE NUMBER: (800) 999-1234 | SOC. SEC. #: 192-76-1544
WHAT IS THE RESPONSIBLE PARTY'S RELATIONSHIP TO THE INSURED? Other

SECONDARY INSURANCE

NAME OF SECONDARY INSURANCE COMPANY:
ADDRESS:
CITY: | STATE: | ZIP CODE:
IDENTIFICATION #: | GROUP NAME AND/OR #:
INSURED PERSON'S NAME (IF DIFFERENT FROM THE RESPONSIBLE PARTY):
ADDRESS (IF DIFFERENT):
CITY: | STATE: | ZIP CODE:
SECONDARY INSURANCE PHONE NUMBER: | SOC. SEC. #:
WHAT IS THE RESPONSIBLE PARTY'S RELATIONSHIP TO THE INSURED?

I hereby consent for Sydney Carrington & Associates, P.A. to use or disclose my health information to carry out treatment, payment, and health care operations. I authorize the use of this signature on all insurance submissions. I understand that I am financially responsible for all charges whether or not paid by the insurance. I acknowledge receipt of the practice's privacy policy.

PATIENT SIGNATURE: Edward R. Glenmore | DATE: 06/02/2008

2. Based on the information found on the patient registration form, add Edward Glenmore as a new patient. Compare your screens to Figures 2-14 through 2-17.

Figure 2-14   Guarantor Information – Glenmore

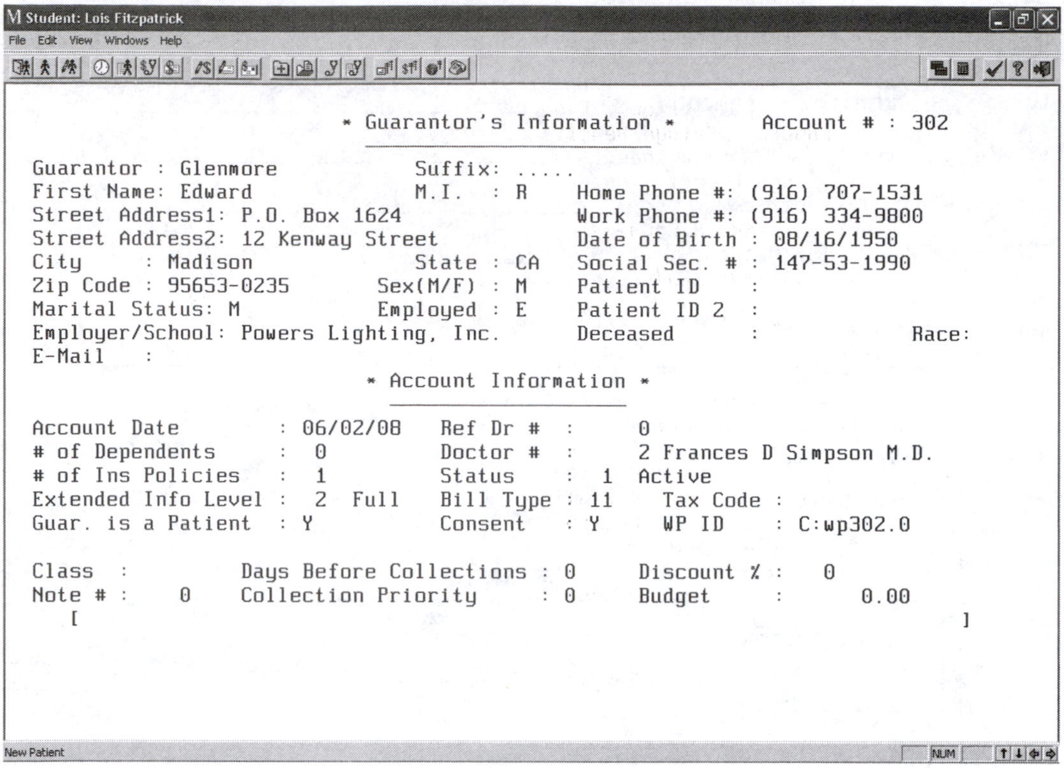

```
M Student: Lois Fitzpatrick                                            _ 🗗 ✕
File  Edit  View  Windows  Help

                      * Guarantor's Information *          Account # : 302

 Guarantor : Glenmore           Suffix: .....
 First Name: Edward             M.I.  : R    Home Phone #: (916) 707-1531
 Street Address1: P.O. Box 1624             Work Phone #: (916) 334-9800
 Street Address2: 12 Kenway Street          Date of Birth : 08/16/1950
 City     : Madison             State : CA  Social Sec. # : 147-53-1990
 Zip Code : 95653-0235          Sex(M/F) : M  Patient ID   :
 Marital Status: M              Employed : E  Patient ID 2 :
 Employer/School: Powers Lighting, Inc.     Deceased      :          Race:
 E-Mail   :
                          * Account Information *

 Account Date      : 06/02/08   Ref Dr # :    0
 # of Dependents   : 0          Doctor # :    2 Frances D Simpson M.D.
 # of Ins Policies : 1          Status   : 1  Active
 Extended Info Level : 2  Full  Bill Type : 11   Tax Code :
 Guar. is a Patient : Y         Consent  : Y   WP ID   : C:wp302.0

 Class  :            Days Before Collections : 0    Discount % :   0
 Note # :    0       Collection Priority    : 0    Budget   :      0.00
   [                                                                    ]


New Patient                                                   NUM    ↑↓⇐⇒
```

Figure 2-15   Guarantor Extended Information – Glenmore

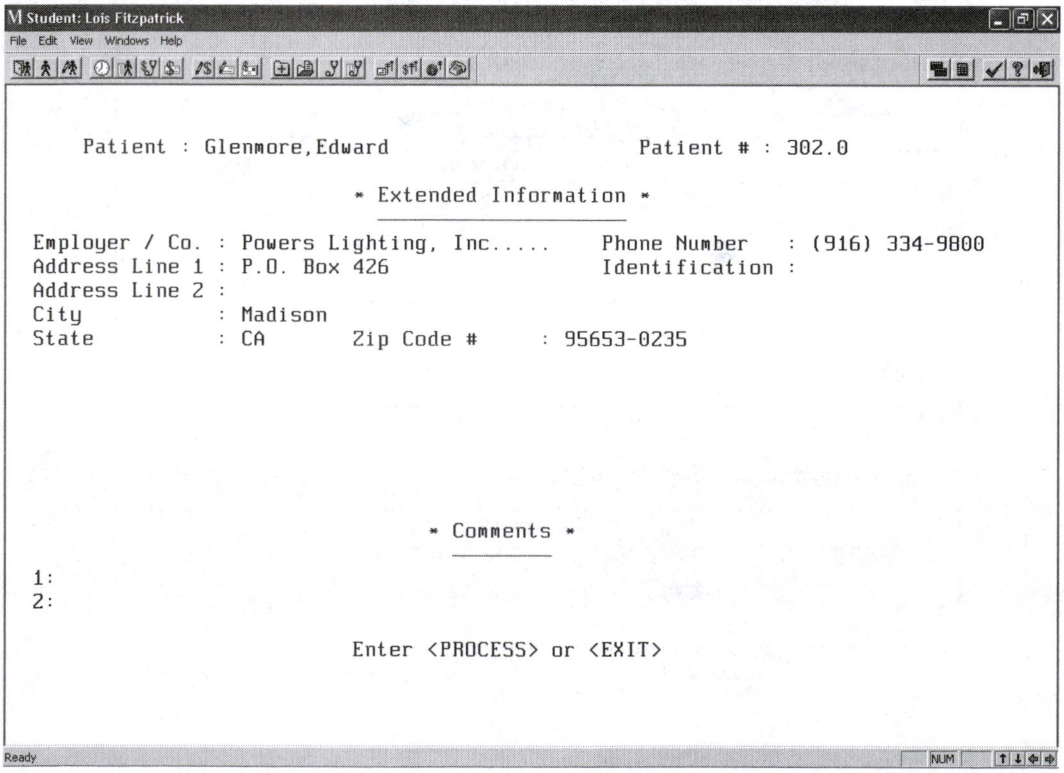

```
M Student: Lois Fitzpatrick                                            _ 🗗 ✕
File  Edit  View  Windows  Help

     Patient : Glenmore,Edward             Patient # : 302.0

                        * Extended Information *

 Employer / Co. : Powers Lighting, Inc.....    Phone Number  : (916) 334-9800
 Address Line 1 : P.O. Box 426                 Identification :
 Address Line 2 :
 City           : Madison
 State          : CA      Zip Code #    : 95653-0235




                          * Comments *

 1:
 2:

                  Enter <PROCESS> or <EXIT>



Ready                                                         NUM    ↑↓⇐⇒
```

Figure 2-16   Insurance Policy – Glenmore

```
M Student: Lois Fitzpatrick                                                    _ ☐ ✕
File  Edit  View  Windows  Help

⊡▥⌖⚙ ⊙ ▦⚉⚐ ⁄⚊⊞  ⊞⚌⚏ ⚑⚑ ⚏⚑⚋⚐        ▤▦ ✓?⚎

    Account #: 302        Insurance Policy Information for 1 of 1     [Glenmore,Edward]
                          ───────────────────────────────────────


    Policyholder    : 0.      [Glenmore, Edward        ]
    Carrier Code    : FRGBEN  [Fringe Benefit Center   ]
    Plan #          : 12      Plan Code:          Form #    : 1    Fmt # : 1
    Plan Name       : Fringe Benefit Center       EMC ID 1  :
    Attention       :                             EMC ID 2  :
    Street Address  : 123 Mission Corners          Deductible:      0.00
    City,State,Zip  : San Mateo        TX   78723  Program   : CI Commercial In
    Phone #         : (800) 999-1234   Class :     Assignment - Dr : Y   Pat : Y
    Group Number    :                              Ins ID #  : 14876PL
    Group Name      : Powers
    Policy Dates - From :         To :             Copay Ext :      Ins Type: C1
            Insured Party #      : 15              Rpt Group :
            Last Name or Company : Powers Lighting, Inc.        Suffix: .....
            First Name, M.I.     : ........... .  Sex   :    DOB :
            Address              : P.O. Box 426
            City,St,Zip          : Madison          CA   95653-0235
            Insured Party ID #   : 192761544        Phone : (916) 334-9800
            Insured's Employer   : Powers Lighting, Inc
            Employer Ins Plan    : Y

        Enter Dependent # of Policyholder, 0 for Guarantor, or '?' for Help


Ready                                                              NUM    ⬆⬇⬅➡
```

Figure 2-17   Insurance Coverage – Glenmore

```
M Student: Lois Fitzpatrick                                                    _ ☐ ✕
File  Edit  View  Windows  Help

⊡▥⌖⚙ ⊙ ▦⚉⚐ ⁄⚊⊞  ⊞⚌⚏ ⚑⚑ ⚏⚑⚋⚐        ▤▦ ✓?⚎

    Patient #: 302.0         Insurance Coverage Priority       [Glenmore,Edward]
                              [Guarantor List]
    Priority    Plan#     Plan Name              IPR          Relation to IPR
    ───────────────────────────────────────────────────────────────────────
    Primary  :  12.0      Fringe Benefit Center  Powers Lighting, Inc    O
    Secondary:
    Third    :  ........
    Fourth   :  ........                                                  .
    Fifth    :  ........                                                  .
    Sixth    :  ........                                                  .
    Seventh  :  ........                                                  .

    [Policies]
    Plan#     Plan Name            Holder     User Note     Insured Party
    ───────────────────────────────────────────────────────────────────────
    12.0   Fringe Benefit Cente  Edward                    Powers Lighting, I
```

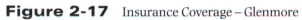

```



        Enter Edward's Relationship to  Powers Lighting, Inc., or '?'
     (S)elf, (W)ife, (H)usband, (C)hild, Special (D)ependent, (P)arent, (O)ther


Ready                                                              NUM    ⬆⬇⬅➡
```

EXERCISE 4: MULTIPLE INSURANCE PLANS

NANCY MONACO; ACCOUNT 303

1. Before attempting data entry, study the patient registration form in Figure 2-18. Answer the following questions.

   a. How many insurances are there? _____

   b. Who is the policyholder of the primary insurance? _____

   Who is the policyholder of the secondary insurance? _____

   c. What is the relationship between the guarantor and the patient? _____

Figure 2-18 Patient Registration – Nancy Monaco

2. Based on the information found on the patient registration form, add Nancy Monaco as a new patient.
Compare your screens to those shown in Figures 2-19 through 2-25.

Figure 2-19   Guarantor Information – Monaco

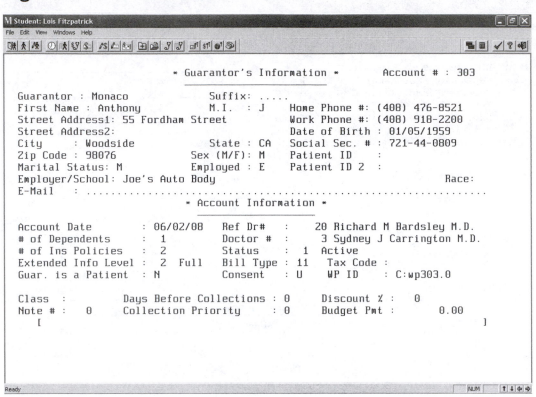

Figure 2-20   Guarantor Extended Information – Monaco

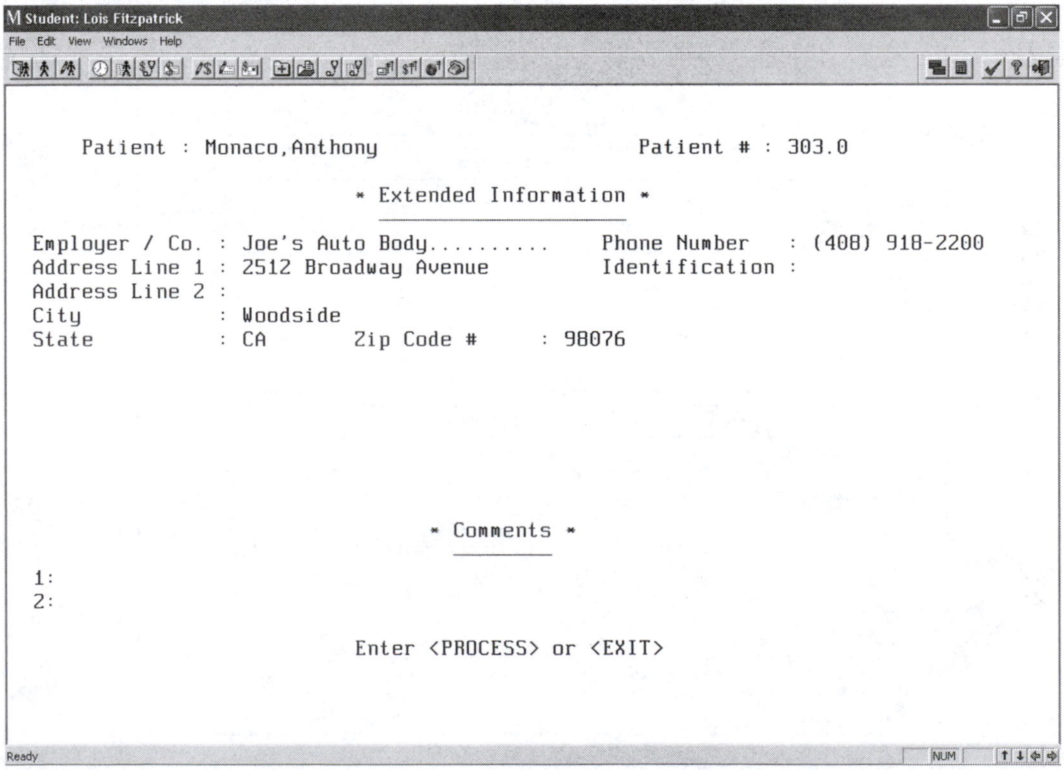

Figure 2-21   Dependent Information – Monaco

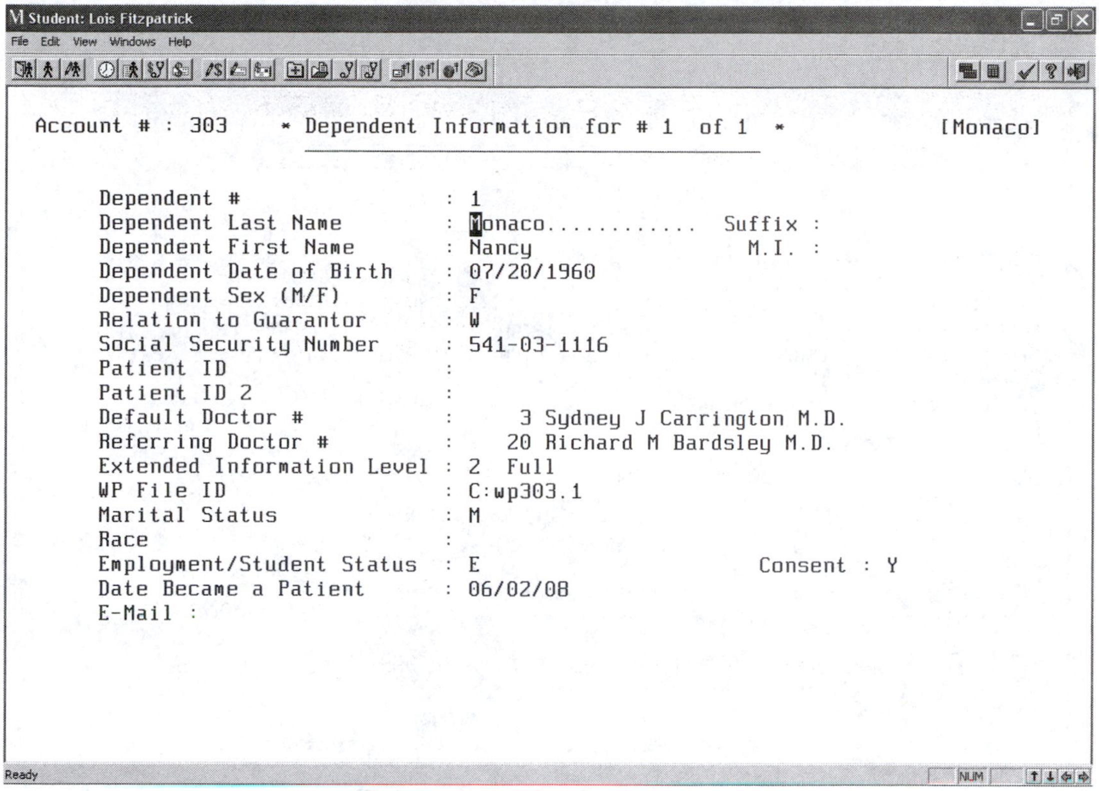

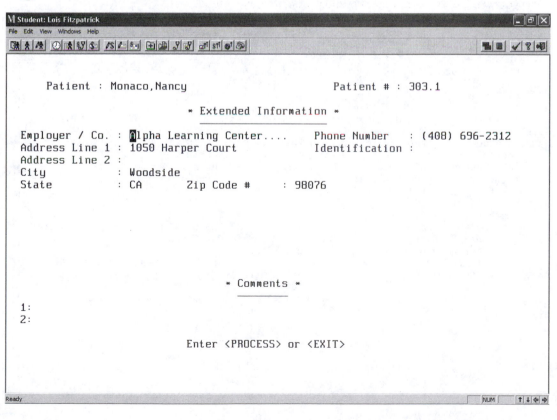

Figure 2-22   Dependent Extended Information – Monaco

Figure 2-23 Insurance Policy 1 – Monaco

```
M Student: Lois Fitzpatrick                                                    _ ☐ ✕
File  Edit  View  Windows  Help

[toolbar icons]                                                      [toolbar icons]

    Account #: 303        Insurance Policy Information for 1 of 2    [Monaco,Anthony ]


    Policyholder    : 0.        [Monaco, Anthony           ]
    Carrier Code    : EPSLON  [Epsilon Life & Casualty  ]
    Plan #          : 5        Plan Code:              Form #   : 1   Fmt # : 1
    Plan Name       : Epsilon Life & Casualty         EMC ID 1 : 44235-13-54849C
    Attention       :                                 EMC ID 2 :
    Street Address  : P.O. Box 189                    Deductible:      300.00
    City,State,Zip  : Macon          GA    31298      Program  : CI Commercial In
    Phone #         : (800) 908-7654   Class : EMC    Assignment – Dr : Y  Pat : Y
    Group Number    : 1298                            Ins ID #  : 18162139
    Group Name      : Group Unnamed                   User Note :
    Policy Dates – From :          To :               Copay Ext :      Ins Type: C1
        Insured Party #          : 0                  Rpt Group :
        Last Name or Company     : Monaco                      Suffix:
        First Name, M.I.         : Anthony      J   Sex  : M  DOB : 01/05/1959
        Address                  : 55 Fordham Street
        City,St,Zip              : Woodside          CA   98076
        Insured Party ID #       : 721-44-0809           Phone : (408) 476-8521
        Insured's Employer       : Joe's Auto Body
        Employer Ins Plan        : Y

        Enter Dependent # of Policyholder, 0 for Guarantor, or '?' for Help



Ready                                                          NUM    ↑↓⇦⇨
```

NOTE: *Insured party numbers are assigned by the computer. The insured party number on your screen may differ from that shown in Figure 2-24.*

Figure 2-24 Insurance Policy 2 – Monaco

```
M Student: Lois Fitzpatrick                                                    _ ☐ ✕
File  Edit  View  Windows  Help

[toolbar icons]                                                      [toolbar icons]

    Account #: 303        Insurance Policy Information for 2 of 2    [Monaco,Anthony ]


    Policyholder    : 1.        [Monaco, Nancy            ]
    Carrier Code    : PANAMC  [Pan American Health Ins. ]
    Plan #          : 7        Plan Code:              Form #   : 1   Fmt # : 1
    Plan Name       : Pan American Health Ins.         EMC ID 1 :
    Attention       :                                 EMC ID 2 :
    Street Address  : 4567 Newberry Rd.               Deductible:        0.00
    City,State,Zip  : Los Angeles      CA   98706     Program  : CI Commercial In
    Phone #         : (213) 456-7654   Class :        Assignment – Dr : Y  Pat : Y
    Group Number    :                                 Ins ID #  : 220627585
    Group Name      : Alpha                           User Note :
    Policy Dates – From :          To :               Copay Ext :      Ins Type: C1
        Insured Party #          : 16                 Rpt Group :
        Last Name or Company     : Monaco                      Suffix:
        First Name, M.I.         : Nancy           Sex  : F  DOB : 07/20/1960
        Address                  : 55 Fordham Street
        City,St,Zip              : Woodside          CA   98076
        Insured Party ID #       : 541-03-1116           Phone : (408) 476-8521
        Insured's Employer       : Alpha Learning Center
        Employer Ins Plan        : Y

        Enter Dependent # of Policyholder, 0 for Guarantor, or '?' for Help



Ready                                                          NUM    ↑↓⇦⇨
```

Figure 2-25 Insurance Coverage – Monaco

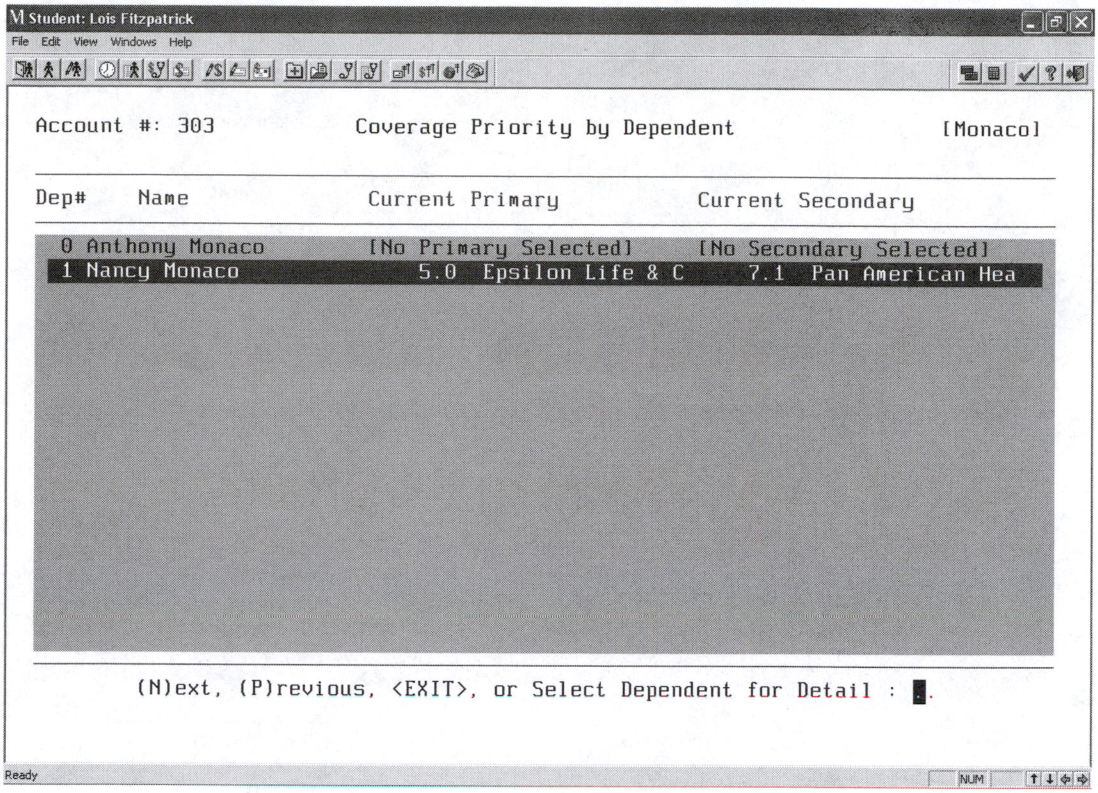

EXERCISE 5: MULTIPLE INSURANCE POLICIES, DIFFERENT INSURED PARTY

VINCENT MONTI; ACCOUNT 304

1. Before attempting data entry, study the patient registration form in Figure 2-26. Answer the following questions.

   a. What is the name of the primary insurance? ______________________

   b. What is the name of the secondary insurance? ______________________

   c. Who is the policyholder for each insurance? ______________________

Figure 2-26 Patient Registration – Vincent Monti

Patient Registration Form

Sydney Carrington & Associates
34 Sycamore Street • Madison, CA 95653

TODAY'S DATE: 06/02/2008

FOR OFFICE USE ONLY	
ACCOUNT NO.:	304
DOCTOR:	#2
BILL TYPE:	11
EXTENDED INFO.:	2

PATIENT INFORMATION

PATIENT LAST NAME: Monti
FIRST NAME: Vincent
MI: A.
SUFFIX:
MAILING ADDRESS:
CITY:
STATE:
ZIP CODE:
SEX (M/F): M
DATE OF BIRTH: 06/23/1968
MARITAL STATUS: Married
SOC. SEC. #: 116-29-1029
HOME PHONE:
RELATIONSHIP TO GUARANTOR: Self
EMPLOYER OR SCHOOL NAME: DLA, Inc.
EMPLOYER OR SCHOOL ADDRESS: 136 Concourse Avenue
CITY: Wallace
STATE: CA
ZIP CODE: 95039
EMPLOYER OR SCHOOL PHONE NUMBER: (916) 971-5381
REFERRED BY: Leland Groves, MD

GUARANTOR INFORMATION

RESPONSIBLE PARTY LAST NAME: Monti
FIRST NAME: Vincent
MI: A.
SEX (M/F): M
DATE OF BIRTH: 06/23/1968
MARITAL STATUS: Married
SOC. SEC. #: 116-29-1029
MAILING ADDRESS: 48 Clermont Road
STREET ADDRESS (IF DIFFERENT):
CITY: Wallace
STATE: CA
ZIP CODE: 95039
(AREA CODE) HOME PHONE: (916) 497-5106
(AREA CODE) WORK PHONE: (916) 971-5381
EMPLOYER NAME: DLA, Inc.
EMPLOYER ADDRESS: 136 Concourse Avenue
CITY: Wallace
STATE: CA
ZIP CODE: 95039

PRIMARY INSURANCE

NAME OF PRIMARY INSURANCE COMPANY: Pan American Health Ins.
ADDRESS: 4567 Newberry Road
CITY: Los Angeles
STATE: CA
ZIP CODE: 98706
IDENTIFICATION #: 1029112753
GROUP NAME AND/OR #:
INSURED PERSON'S NAME (IF DIFFERENT FROM THE RESPONSIBLE PARTY): Sandra B. Monti
ADDRESS (IF DIFFERENT): Same
CITY: Same
STATE:
ZIP CODE:
PRIMARY INSURANCE PHONE NUMBER: (213) 456-7654
SOC. SEC. #: 012-44-0112
WHAT IS THE RESPONSIBLE PARTY'S RELATIONSHIP TO THE INSURED? Husband

SECONDARY INSURANCE

NAME OF SECONDARY INSURANCE COMPANY: Epsilon Life & Casualty
ADDRESS: P.O. Box 189
CITY: Macon
STATE: GA
ZIP CODE: 31298
IDENTIFICATION #: 01121616
GROUP NAME AND/OR #: DLA
INSURED PERSON'S NAME (IF DIFFERENT FROM THE RESPONSIBLE PARTY): Vincent A. Monti
ADDRESS (IF DIFFERENT): Same
CITY: Same
STATE:
ZIP CODE:
SECONDARY INSURANCE PHONE NUMBER: (800) 908-7654
SOC. SEC. #: 116-29-1029
WHAT IS THE RESPONSIBLE PARTY'S RELATIONSHIP TO THE INSURED? Self

I hereby consent for Sydney Carrington & Associates, P.A. to use or disclose my health information to carry out treatment, payment, and health care operations. I authorize the use of this signature on all insurance submissions. I understand that I am financially responsible for all charges whether or not paid by the insurance. I acknowledge receipt of the practice's privacy policy.

PATIENT SIGNATURE: Vincent A. Monti
DATE: 06/02/2008

2. Based on the information found on the patient registration form, add Vincent Monti as a new patient. Compare your screens to Figures 2-27 through 2-31.

REMINDER: *If a city does not appear in the HOME menu, press ESCAPE and type the information in the field.*

Figure 2-27   Guarantor Information – Monti

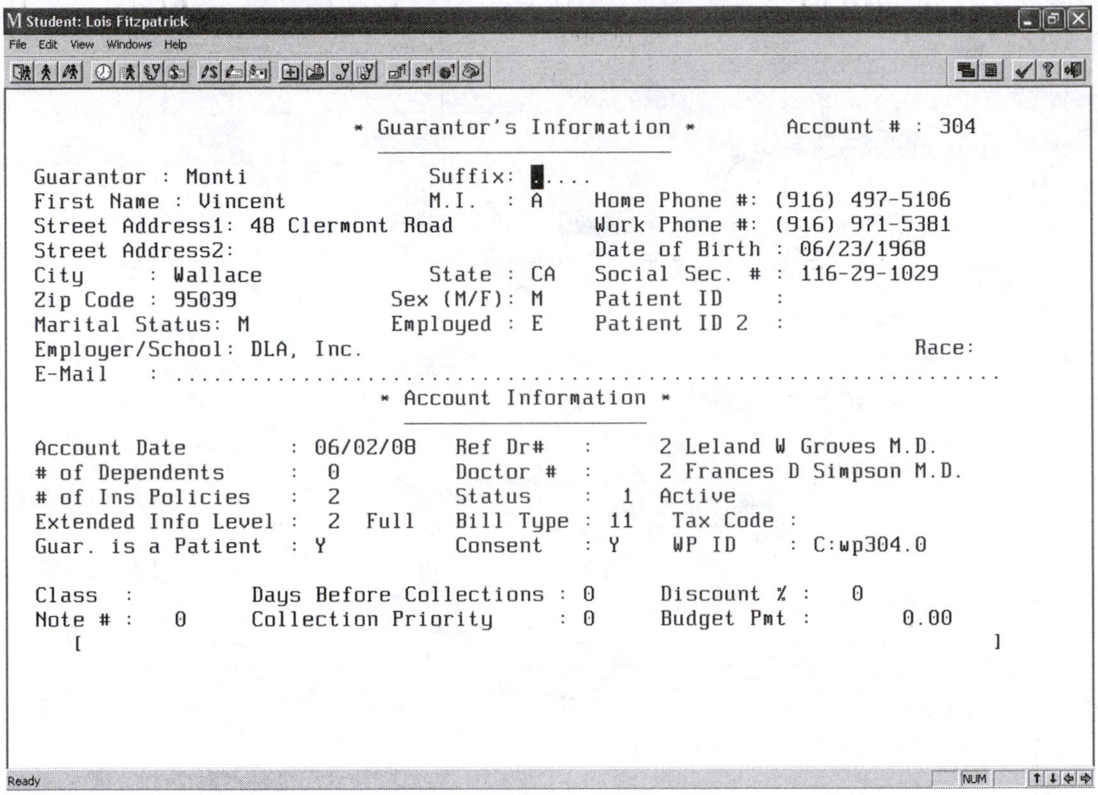

Figure 2-28   Extended Information – Monti

```
M Student: Lois Fitzpatrick                                                    _ □ X
File  Edit  View  Windows  Help
[toolbar icons]                                                    [toolbar icons]



       Patient : Monti,Vincent                    Patient # : 304.0

                         * Extended Information *
                         _____

   Employer / Co. : DLA, Inc................    Phone Number   : (916) 971-5381
   Address Line 1 : 136 Concourse Avenue       Identification :
   Address Line 2 :
   City           : Wallace
   State          : CA      Zip Code #    : 95039




                              * Comments *
                              _____

   1:
   2:

                      Enter <PROCESS> or <EXIT>




Ready                                                              NUM    ↑↓◄►
```

NOTE: *Insured party numbers are assigned by the computer. The number assigned in Exercise 5 may differ from that shown in Figure 2-29.*

Figure 2-29   Insurance Policy 1 – Monti

```
M Student: Lois Fitzpatrick                                                    _ □ X
File  Edit  View  Windows  Help
[toolbar icons]                                                    [toolbar icons]


   Account #: 304       Insurance Policy Information for 1 of 2   [Monti,Vincent  ]


   Policyholder      : 0.      [Monti, Vincent        ]
   Carrier Code      : PANAMC  [Pan American Health Ins. ]
   Plan #            : 7        Plan Code:          Form #    : 1    Fmt # : 1
   Plan Name         : Pan American Health Ins.     EMC ID 1 :
   Attention         :                              EMC ID 2 :
   Street Address : 4567 Newberry Rd.               Deductible:      0.00
   City,State,Zip : Los Angeles      CA   98706     Program   : CI Commercial In
   Phone #        : (213) 456-7654    Class :       Assignment - Dr : Y  Pat : Y
   Group Number   :                                 Ins ID #  : 1029112753
   Group Name     : Alpha                           User Note :
   Policy Dates - From :          To :              Copay Ext :       Ins Type: C1
           Insured Party #     : 17                 Rpt Group :
           Last Name or Company : Monti                        Suffix:
           First Name, M.I.    : Sandra       B  Sex   : F  DOB :
           Address             : 48 Clermont Road
           City,St,Zip         : Wallace         CA   95039
           Insured Party ID #  : 012440112          Phone : (916) 497-5106
           Insured's Employer  :
           Employer Ins Plan   :

           Enter Dependent # of Policyholder, 0 for Guarantor, or '?' for Help


Ready                                                              NUM    ↑↓◄►
```

Figure 2-30 Insurance Policy 2 – Monti

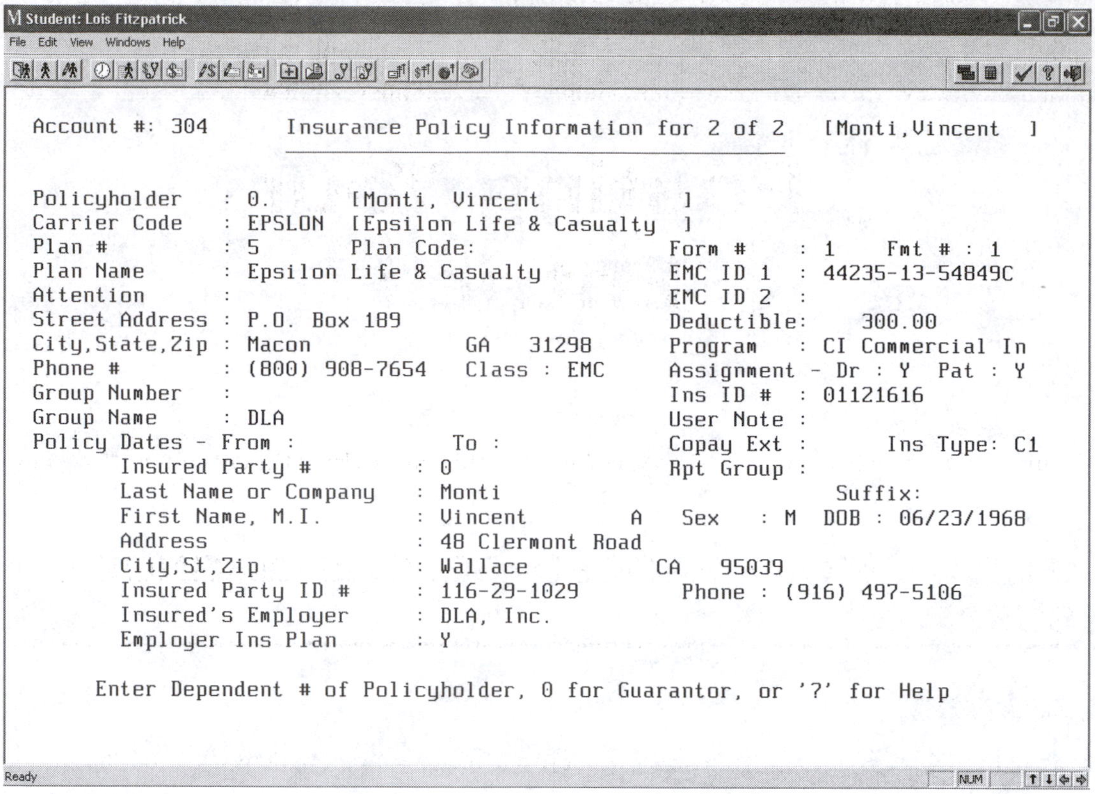

Figure 2-31 Insurance Coverage – Monti

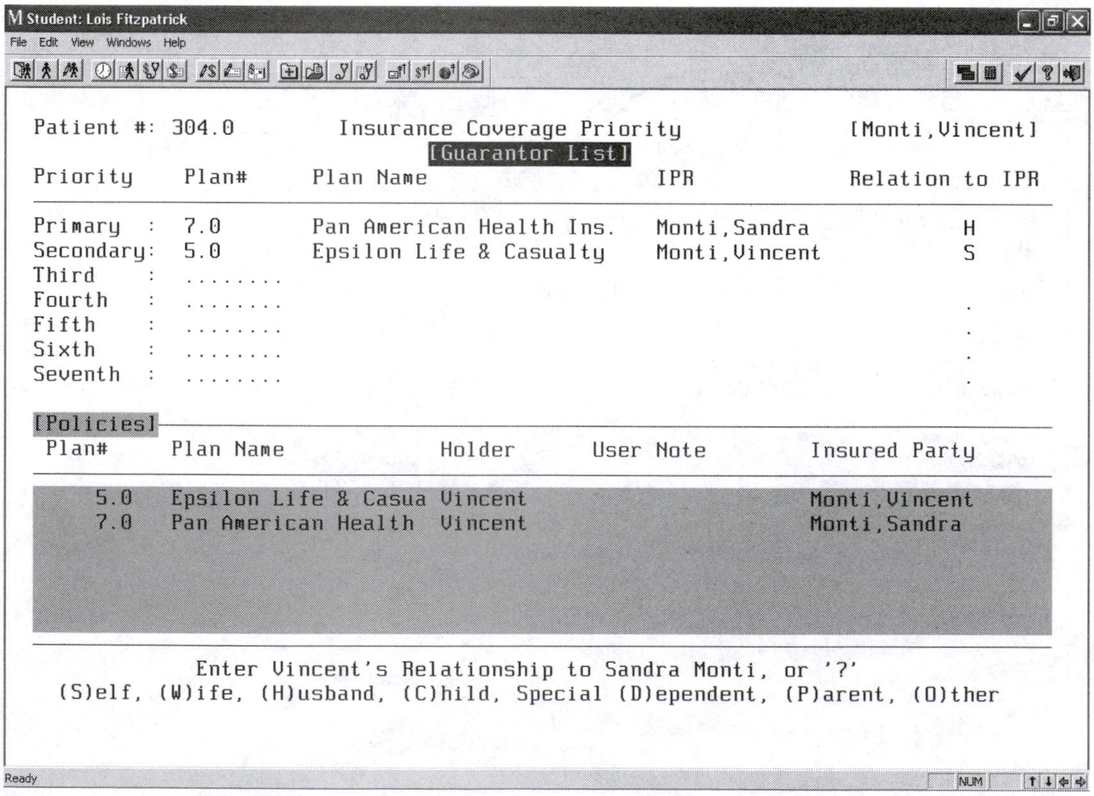

U N I T 3

Posting Your Entries

In the unit exercises that follow, you will be posting procedure entries from the encounter forms provided.

EXERCISE 1: ONE PROCEDURE, ONE DIAGNOSIS, NO INSURANCE

JUAN PEREZ

GOAL(S): In this exercise, you will enter a procedure and diagnosis for a patient with no insurance.

1. Before posting your entry, study the encounter form in Figure 3-1. Answer the following questions.

   a. Who is the patient? _____

   b. What is the voucher number on the encounter form? _____

   c. Which doctor saw the patient? _____

   d. How many procedures were completed at this visit? _____

   e. How many diagnoses are listed? _____

Figure 3-1   Encounter Form – Perez

Sydney Carrington & Associates P.A.
34 Sycamore Street Suite 300
Madison, CA 95653

Date: 06/02/2008   Voucher No.: 4030

Time:

Patient: Juan Perez   Patient No: 309.0
Guarantor: Doctor: 3 – S. Carrington

☐ CPT	DESCRIPTION	FEE
OFFICE/HOSPITAL CONSULTS		
☐ 99201	Office New:Focused Hx-Exam	___
☐ 99202	Office New:Expanded Hx.Exam	___
☐ 99211	Office Estb:Min./None Hx-Exa	___
☐ 99212	Office Estb:Focused Hx-Exam	___
☐ 99213	Office Estb:Expanded Hx-Exa	___
☒ 99214	Office Estb:Detailed Hx-Exa	___
☐ 99215	Office Estb:Comprhn Hx-Exam	___
☐ 99221	Hosp. Initial:Comprh Hx-	___
☐ 99223	Hosp. Ini:Comprh Hx-Exam/Hi	___
☐ 99231	Hosp. Subsequent: S-Fwd	___
☐ 99232	Hosp. Subsequent: Comprhn Hx	___
☐ 99233	Hosp. Subsequent: Ex/Hi	___
☐ 99238	Hospital Visit Discharge Ex	___
☐ 99371	Telephone Consult - Simple	___
☐ 99372	Telephone Consult - Intermed	___
☐ 99373	Telephone Consult - Complex	___
☐ 90840	Counseling - 25 minutes	___
☐ 90806	Counseling - 50 minutes	___
☐ 90865	Counseling - Special Interview	___
IMMUNIZATIONS/INJECTIONS		
☐ 90585	BCG Vaccine	___
☐ 90659	Influenza Virus Vaccine	___
☐ 90701	Immunization-DTP	___
☐ 90702	DT Vaccine	___
☐ 90703	Tetanus Toxoids	___
☐ 90732	Pneumococcal Vaccine	___
☐ 90746	Hepatitis B Vaccine	___
☐ 90749	Immunization: Unlisted	___

☐ CPT	DESCRIPTION	FEE
LABORATORY/RADIOLOGY		
☐ 81000	Urinalysis	___
☐ 81002	Urinalysis; Pregnancy Test	___
☐ 82951	Glucose Tolerance Test	___
☐ 84478	Triglycerides	___
☐ 84550	Uric Acid: Blood Chemistry	___
☐ 84830	Ovulation Test	___
☐ 85014	Hematocrit	___
☐ 85032	Hemogram, Complete Blood Wk	___
☐ 86403	Particle Agglutination Test	___
☐ 86485	Skin Test; Candida	___
☐ 86580	TB Intradermal Test	___
☐ 86585	TB Tine Test	___
☐ 87070	Culture	___
☐ 70190	X-Ray; Optic Foramina	___
☐ 70210	X-Ray Sinuses Complete	___
☐ 71010	Radiological Exam Ent Spine	___
☐ 71020	X-Ray Chest Pa & Lat	___
☐ 72050	X-Ray Spine, Cerv (4 views)	___
☐ 72090	X-Ray Spine; Scoliosis Ex	___
☐ 72110	Spine, lumbosacral; a/p & Lat	___
☐ 73030	Shoulder-Comp, min w/ 2vws	___
☐ 73070	Elbow, anteropost & later vws	___
☐ 73120	X-Ray; Hand, 2 views	___
☐ 73560	X-Ray, Knee, 1 or 2 views	___
☐ 74022	X-Ray; Abdomen, Complete	___
☐ 75552	Cardiac Magnetic Res Img	___
☐ 76020	X-Ray; Bone Age Studies	___
☐ 77054	Mammary Ductogram Complete	___
☐ 78465	Myocardial Perfusion Img	___

☐ CPT	DESCRIPTION	FEE
PROCEDURES/TESTS		
☐ 00452	Anesthesia for Rad Surgery	___
☐ 11100	Skin Biopsy	___
☐ 15852	Dressing Change	___
☐ 29075	Cast Appl. - Lower Arm	___
☐ 29530	Strapping of Knee	___
☐ 29705	Removal/Revis of Cast w/Exa	___
☐ 53670	Catheterization Incl. Suppl	___
☐ 57452	Colposcopy	___
☐ 57505	ECC	___
☐ 69420	Myringotomy	___
☐ 92081	Visual Field Examination	___
☐ 92100	Serial Tonometry Exam	___
☐ 92120	Tonography	___
☐ 92552	Pure Tone Audiometry	___
☐ 92567	Tympanometry	___
☐ 93000	Electrocardiogram	___
☐ 93015	Exercise Stress Test (ETT)	___
☐ 93017	ETT Tracing Only	___
☐ 93040	Electrocardiogram - Rhythm	___
☐ 96100	Psychological Testing	___
☐ 99000	Specimen Handling	___
☐ 99058	Office Emergency Care	___
☐ 99070	Surgical Tray - Misc.	___
☐ 99080	Special Reports of Med Rec	___
☐ 99195	Phlebotomy	___
☐	_____	___
☐	_____	___
☐	_____	___

☐	ICD-9 CODE DIAGNOSIS	
☐ 009.0	Infect. colitis, enteritis, & gastroenteritis	
☐ 133.0	Scabies	
☐ 174.9	Breast Cancer, Female, Unspecified	
☐ 185	Malignant neoplasm of prostate	
☐ 250.00	Diabetes Mellitus w/o mention of Complication	
☐ 272.4	Hyperlipidemia	
☐ 282.5	Anemia, Sickle-cell Trait	
☐ 282.60	Sickle-cell disease, unspecified	
☐ 285.9	Anemia, Unspecified	
☐ 300.4	Dysthymic disorder	
☐ 340	Multiple Sclerosis	
☐ 342.90	Hemiplegia - Unspec.	
☐ 346.90	Migraine, unspecified	
☐ 352.9	Unspecified disorder of cranial nerves	
☐ 354.0	Carpal Tunnel Syndrome	
☐ 355.0	Sciatic Nerve Root Lesion	
☐ 366.9	Cataract	
☐ 386.00	Menier's disease, unspecified	
☒ 401.1	Essential Hypertension, Benign	
☐ 414.9	Ischemic Heart Disease	
☐ 428.0	Congestive Heart Failure (CHF), unspecified	

☐	ICD-9 CODE DIAGNOSIS	
☐ 435.0	Basilar Artery Syndrome	
☐ 440.0	Atherosclerosis	
☐ 442.81	Carotid Artery	
☐ 460	Common Cold (Acute Nasopharyngitis)	
☐ 461.9	Acute Sinusitis	
☐ 474.00	Chronic Tonsillitis & Adenoiditis	
☐ 477.9	Allergic Rhinitis, Cause Unspecified	
☐ 487.0	Influenza with pneumonia	
☐ 496	Chronic Airway Obstruction	
☐ 522.0	Pulpitis	
☐ 524.60	Temporo-Mandibular Joint Disorder - Unspec.	
☐ 536.8	Stomach Pain	
☐ 553.3	Hiatal Hernia	
☐ 564.1	Spastic Colon	
☐ 574.40	Chronic Hepatitis, Unspecified	
☐ 571.5	Cirrhosis of Liver w/o mention of alcohol	
☐ 573.3	Hepatitis	
☐ 575.2	Obstruction of Gallbladder	
☐ 648.20	Anemia - Compl. Pregnancy	
☐ 715.90	Osteoarthritis - Unspec.	
☐ 721.3	Lumbar Osteo/Spondylarthrit	

☐	ICD-9 CODE DIAGNOSIS	
☐ 724.2	Pain: Lower Back	
☐ 727.67	Rupture of Achilles Tendon	
☐ 780.1	Hallucinations	
☐ 780.3	Convulsions, Other	
☐ 780.50	Sleep Disturbances, Unspecified	
☐ 783.0	Anorexia	
☐ 783.1	Abnormal Weight Gain	
☐ 783.21	Abnormal Weight Loss	
☐ 823.80	Fractured Tibia	
☐ 823.81	Fractured Fibula	
☐ 831.00	Dislocated Shoulder, Closed, Unspecified	
☐ 835.00	Dislocated Hip, Closed, Unspecified	
☐ 842.00	Sprained Wrist, Unspecified Site	
☐ 845.00	Sprained Ankle, Unspecified Site	
☐ 919.5	Insect Bite, Nonvenomous	
☐ 921.1	Contus Eyelid/Perioc Area	
☐ v16.3	Fam. Hist of Breast Cancer	
☐ v17.4	Fam. Hist of Cardiovasc Dis	
☐ v20.2	Well Child	
☐ v22.0	Pregnancy - First Normal	
☐ v22.1	Pregnancy - Normal	

Previous Balance	Today's Charges	Total Due	Amount Paid	New Balance
___	___	___	___	___

Follow Up

PRN _____ Weeks _____ Months _____ Units _____

Next Appointment Date: Time:

I hereby authorize release of any information acquired in the course of
examination or treatment and allow a photocopy of my signature to be used.

_____

2. Based on the information found on the encounter form, enter the procedure and diagnosis for Juan
   Perez. Compare your screen to Figure 3-2.

Figure 3-2   Procedure Entry – Perez

```
M Student: Lois Fitzpatrick                                                    _ 🗗 ✕
File  Edit  View  Windows  Help
🔲▮ ▮ ▮  🕐 ▮▮ ▮ 💲 /▮▮▮▮  ⊞▮ 🗐 ▮▮  ▮ st ▮▮                                   ▮▮ ▮ ✓ ? ▮

  Patient #: 309.0     [Juan Perez                         ]      Dept.    : 0
  Voucher #: ▮030..            Doctor # :   3 Carrington M.D., S  Location :
                               Supervisor:  3 Carrington M.D., S
  Dates     P.O.S.  Procedure   Modifier Diag. 1-4    Units       Charges   T.O.S.

  06/02/08  3       99214                              1.00   $      50.00  1

 |Office Estb:Detailed Hx-Exam/Modera|401.1       Essential Hypertension, Benign|
  Comment:                            |
                                      |.........
                                      |.........
  Ins: Primary#: 0.0        Assign: .    Secondary#: .......    EMC Billable: .




Ready                                                               NUM    ▮ ▮ ⬅ ➡
```

EXERCISE 2: ONE PROCEDURE, ONE DIAGNOSIS, ONE INSURANCE

CATHERINE VIAJO

GOAL(S): In this exercise, you will enter a procedure and diagnosis for a patient with one insurance.

1. Before posting your entry, study the encounter form in Figure 3-3. Answer the following questions.

   a. Who is the patient? _____

   b. What is the voucher number on the encounter form? _____

   c. Which doctor saw the patient? _____

   d. How many procedures were completed at this visit? _____

   e. How many diagnoses are listed? _____

Figure 3-3 Encounter Form – Viajo

Sydney Carrington & Associates P.A.
34 Sycamore Street Suite 300
Madison, CA 95653

Date: 06/02/2008   Voucher No.: 4031

Time:

Patient: Catherine Viajo   Patient No: 305.0
Guarantor: Doctor: 3 - S. Carrington

☐	CPT	DESCRIPTION	FEE
		OFFICE/HOSPITAL CONSULTS	
☐	99201	Office New:Focused Hx-Exam	
☐	99202	Office New:Expanded Hx.Exam	
☐	99211	Office Estb:Min./None Hx-Exa	
☐	99212	Office Estb:Focused Hx-Exam	
☒	99213	Office Estb:Expanded Hx-Exa	
☐	99214	Office Estb:Detailed Hx-Exa	
☐	99215	Office Estb:Comprhn Hx-Exam	
☐	99221	Hosp. Initial:Comprh Hx-	
☐	99223	Hosp. Ini:Comprh Hx-Exam/Hi	
☐	99231	Hosp. Subsequent: S-Fwd	
☐	99232	Hosp. Subsequent: Comprhn Hx	
☐	99233	Hosp. Subsequent: Ex/Hi	
☐	99238	Hospital Visit Discharge Ex	
☐	99371	Telephone Consult - Simple	
☐	99372	Telephone Consult - Intermed	
☐	99373	Telephone Consult - Complex	
☐	90840	Counseling - 25 minutes	
☐	90806	Counseling - 50 minutes	
☐	90865	Counseling - Special Interview	
		IMMUNIZATIONS/INJECTIONS	
☐	90585	BCG Vaccine	
☐	90659	Influenza Virus Vaccine	
☐	90701	Immunization-DTP	
☐	90702	DT Vaccine	
☐	90703	Tetanus Toxoids	
☐	90732	Pneumococcal Vaccine	
☐	90746	Hepatitis B Vaccine	
☐	90749	Immunization: Unlisted	

☐	CPT	DESCRIPTION	FEE
		LABORATORY/RADIOLOGY	
☐	81000	Urinalysis	
☐	81002	Urinalysis; Pregnancy Test	
☐	82951	Glucose Tolerance Test	
☐	84478	Triglycerides	
☐	84550	Uric Acid: Blood Chemistry	
☐	84830	Ovulation Test	
☐	85014	Hematocrit	
☐	85032	Hemogram, Complete Blood Wk	
☐	86403	Particle Agglutination Test	
☐	86485	Skin Test; Candida	
☐	86580	TB Intradermal Test	
☐	86585	TB Tine Test	
☐	87070	Culture	
☐	70190	X-Ray; Optic Foramina	
☐	70210	X-Ray Sinuses Complete	
☐	71010	Radiological Exam Ent Spine	
☐	71020	X-Ray Chest Pa & Lat	
☐	72050	X-Ray Spine, Cerv (4 views)	
☐	72090	X-Ray Spine; Scoliosis Ex	
☐	72110	Spine, lumbosacral; a/p & Lat	
☐	73030	Shoulder-Comp, min w/ 2vws	
☐	73070	Elbow, anteropost & later vws	
☐	73120	X-Ray; Hand, 2 views	
☐	73560	X-Ray, Knee, 1 or 2 views	
☐	74022	X-Ray; Abdomen, Complete	
☐	75552	Cardiac Magnetic Res Img	
☐	76020	X-Ray; Bone Age Studies	
☐	77054	Mammary Ductogram Complete	
☐	78465	Myocardial Perfusion Img	

☐	CPT	DESCRIPTION	FEE
		PROCEDURES/TESTS	
☐	00452	Anesthesia for Rad Surgery	
☐	11100	Skin Biopsy	
☐	15852	Dressing Change	
☐	29075	Cast Appl. - Lower Arm	
☐	29530	Strapping of Knee	
☐	29705	Removal/Revis of Cast w/Exa	
☐	53670	Catheterization Incl. Suppl	
☐	57452	Colposcopy	
☐	57505	ECC	
☐	69420	Myringotomy	
☐	92081	Visual Field Examination	
☐	92100	Serial Tonometry Exam	
☐	92120	Tonography	
☐	92552	Pure Tone Audiometry	
☐	92567	Tympanometry	
☐	93000	Electrocardiogram	
☐	93015	Exercise Stress Test (ETT)	
☐	93017	ETT Tracing Only	
☐	93040	Electrocardiogram - Rhythm	
☐	96100	Psychological Testing	
☐	99000	Specimen Handling	
☐	99058	Office Emergency Care	
☐	99070	Surgical Tray - Misc.	
☐	99080	Special Reports of Med Rec	
☐	99195	Phlebotomy	
☐			
☐			
☐			

☐	ICD-9 CODE DIAGNOSIS	
☐	009.0	Infect. colitis, enteritis, & gastroenteritis
☐	133.0	Scabies
☐	174.9	Breast Cancer, Female, Unspecified
☐	185	Malignant neoplasm of prostate
☐	250.00	Diabetes Mellitus w/o mention of Complication
☐	272.4	Hyperlipidemia
☐	282.5	Anemia, Sickle-cell Trait
☐	282.60	Sickle-cell disease, unspecified
☐	285.9	Anemia, Unspecified
☐	300.4	Dysthymic disorder
☐	340	Multiple Sclerosis
☐	342.90	Hemiplegia - Unspec.
☒	346.90	Migraine, unspecified
☐	352.9	Unspecified disorder of cranial nerves
☐	354.0	Carpal Tunnel Syndrome
☐	355.0	Sciatic Nerve Root Lesion
☐	366.9	Cataract
☐	386.00	Menier's disease, unspecified
☐	401.1	Essential Hypertension, Benign
☐	414.9	Ischemic Heart Disease
☐	428.0	Congestive Heart Failure (CHF), unspecified

☐	ICD-9 CODE DIAGNOSIS	
☐	435.0	Basilar Artery Syndrome
☐	440.0	Atherosclerosis
☐	442.81	Carotid Artery
☐	460	Common Cold (Acute Nasopharyngitis)
☐	461.9	Acute Sinusitis
☐	474.00	Chronic Tonsillitis & Adenoiditis
☐	477.9	Allergic Rhinitis, Cause Unspecified
☐	487.0	Influenza with pneumonia
☐	496	Chronic Airway Obstruction
☐	522.0	Pulpitis
☐	524.60	Temporo-Mandibular Joint Disorder - Unspec.
☐	536.8	Stomach Pain
☐	553.3	Hiatal Hernia
☐	564.1	Spastic Colon
☐	574.40	Chronic Hepatitis, Unspecified
☐	571.5	Cirrhosis of Liver w/o mention of alcohol
☐	573.3	Hepatitis
☐	575.2	Obstruction of Gallbladder
☐	648.20	Anemia - Compl. Pregnancy
☐	715.90	Osteoarthritis - Unspec.
☐	721.3	Lumbar Osteo/Spondylarthrit

☐	ICD-9 CODE DIAGNOSIS	
☐	724.2	Pain: Lower Back
☐	727.67	Rupture of Achilles Tendon
☐	780.1	Hallucinations
☐	780.3	Convulsions, Other
☐	780.50	Sleep Disturbances, Unspecified
☐	783.0	Anorexia
☐	783.1	Abnormal Weight Gain
☐	783.21	Abnormal Weight Loss
☐	823.80	Fractured Tibia
☐	823.81	Fractured Fibula
☐	831.00	Dislocated Shoulder, Closed, Unspecified
☐	835.00	Dislocated Hip, Closed, Unspecified
☐	842.00	Sprained Wrist, Unspecified Site
☐	845.00	Sprained Ankle, Unspecified Site
☐	919.5	Insect Bite, Nonvenomous
☐	921.1	Contus Eyelid/Perioc Area
☐	v16.3	Fam. Hist of Breast Cancer
☐	v17.4	Fam. Hist of Cardiovasc Dis
☐	v20.2	Well Child
☐	v22.0	Pregnancy - First Normal
☐	v22.1	Pregnancy - Normal

Previous Balance	Today's Charges	Total Due	Amount Paid	New Balance

Follow Up

PRN _____ Weeks _____ Months _____ Units _____

Next Appointment Date: _____   Time: _____

I hereby authorize release of any information acquired in the course of
examination or treatment and allow a photocopy of my signature to be used.

_____

2. Based on the information found on the encounter form, enter the procedure and diagnosis for Catherine Viajo. Compare your screen to Figure 3-4.

Figure 3-4 Procedure Entry – Viajo

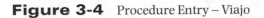

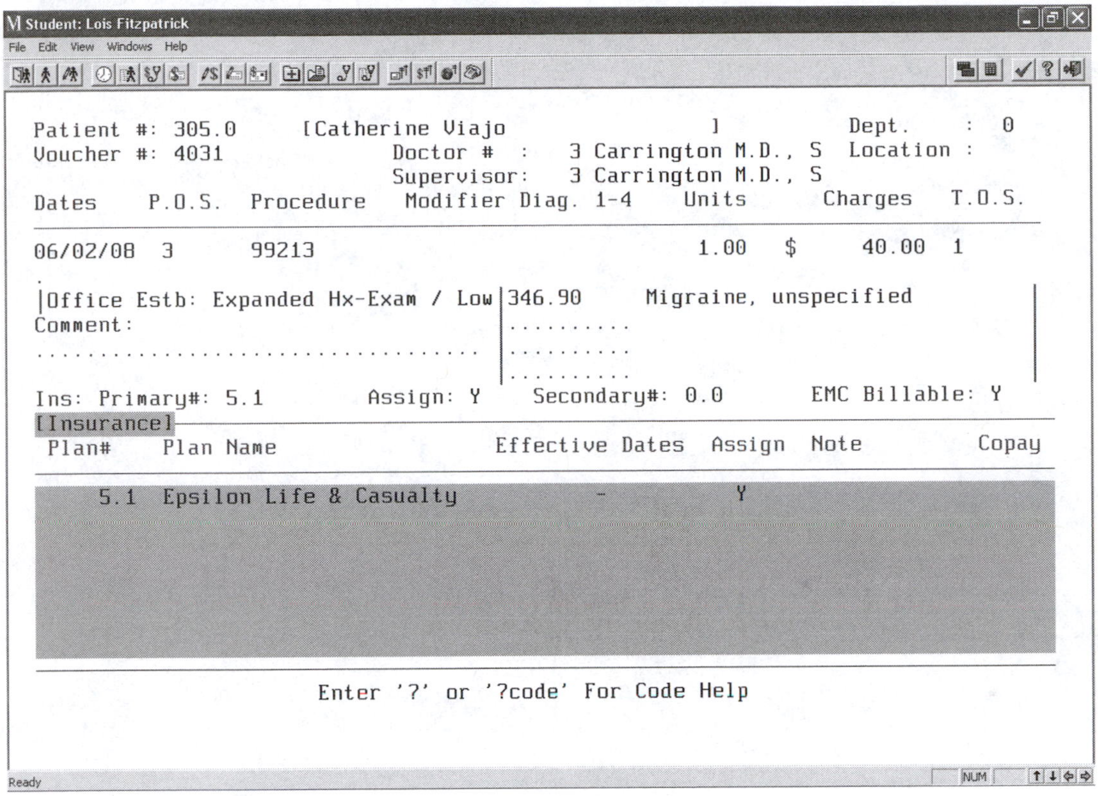

```
M Student: Lois Fitzpatrick                                              _ ☐ X
File  Edit  View  Windows  Help
  ▯▯ ▯ ▯ ⊙ ▯▯ ▯ ▯▯▯ ▯▯▯ ▯▯ ▯ ▯▯ ▯▯                          ▯ ▯ ✓ ? ▯

   Patient #: 305.0     [Catherine Viajo              ]        Dept.    :  0
   Voucher #: 4031             Doctor # :   3 Carrington M.D., S  Location :
                               Supervisor:   3 Carrington M.D., S
   Dates     P.O.S.  Procedure   Modifier Diag. 1-4   Units      Charges  T.O.S.

   06/02/08  3        99213                           1.00  $      40.00  1

   |Office Estb: Expanded Hx-Exam / Low|346.90     Migraine, unspecified
   Comment:                             | . . . . . . . . . .
   . . . . . . . . . . . . . . . . . . . . . . . . . . . | . . . . . . . . . .
                                        | . . . . . . . . . .
   Ins: Primary#: 5.1        Assign: Y     Secondary#: 0.0      EMC Billable: Y
   [Insurance]
    Plan#    Plan Name                Effective Dates  Assign  Note      Copay

     5.1  Epsilon Life & Casualty              -          Y



                        Enter '?' or '?code' For Code Help


 Ready                                                       NUM    ↑ ↓ ⇐ ⇒
```

EXERCISE 3: MULTIPLE PROCEDURES, ONE DIAGNOSIS, ONE INSURANCE

JOHN WYATT

GOAL(S): In this exercise, you will enter multiple procedures and a single diagnosis for a patient with insurance.

1. Before posting your entry, study the encounter form in Figure 3-5. Answer the following questions.

   a. Who is the patient? _____

   b. What is the voucher number on the encounter form? _____

   c. Which doctor saw the patient? _____

   d. How many procedures were completed at this visit? _____

   e. How many diagnoses are listed? _____

Figure 3-5   Encounter Form – Wyatt

Sydney Carrington & Associates P.A.
34 Sycamore Street Suite 300
Madison, CA 95653

Date: 06/02/2008

Time:

Patient: John Wyatt
Guarantor:

Voucher No.:   4032

Patient No: 307.0
Doctor: 1 - J. Monroe

	CPT	DESCRIPTION	FEE
	OFFICE/HOSPITAL CONSULTS		
☐	99201	Office New:Focused Hx-Exam	___
☐	99202	Office New:Expanded Hx.Exam	___
☐	99211	Office Estb:Min./None Hx-Exa	___
☐	99212	Office Estb:Focused Hx-Exam	___
☒	99213	Office Estb:Expanded Hx-Exa	___
☐	99214	Office Estb:Detailed Hx-Exa	___
☐	99215	Office Estb:Comprhn Hx-Exam	___
☐	99221	Hosp. Initial:Comprh Hx-	___
☐	99223	Hosp. Ini:Comprh Hx-Exam/Hi	___
☐	99231	Hosp. Subsequent: S-Fwd	___
☐	99232	Hosp. Subsequent: Comprhn Hx	___
☐	99233	Hosp. Subsequent: Ex/Hi	___
☐	99238	Hospital Visit Discharge Ex	___
☐	99371	Telephone Consult - Simple	___
☐	99372	Telephone Consult - Intermed	___
☐	99373	Telephone Consult - Complex	___
☐	90840	Counseling - 25 minutes	___
☐	90806	Counseling - 50 minutes	___
☐	90865	Counseling - Special Interview	___
	IMMUNIZATIONS/INJECTIONS		
☐	90585	BCG Vaccine	___
☐	90659	Influenza Virus Vaccine	___
☐	90701	Immunization-DTP	___
☐	90702	DT Vaccine	___
☐	90703	Tetanus Toxoids	___
☐	90732	Pneumococcal Vaccine	___
☐	90746	Hepatitis B Vaccine	___
☐	90749	Immunization: Unlisted	___

	CPT	DESCRIPTION	FEE
	LABORATORY/RADIOLOGY		
☐	81000	Urinalysis	___
☐	81002	Urinalysis; Pregnancy Test	___
☐	82951	Glucose Tolerance Test	___
☐	84478	Triglycerides	___
☐	84550	Uric Acid: Blood Chemistry	___
☐	84830	Ovulation Test	___
☒	85014	Hematocrit	___
☒	85032	Hemogram, Complete Blood Wk	___
☐	86403	Particle Agglutination Test	___
☐	86485	Skin Test; Candida	___
☐	86580	TB Intradermal Test	___
☐	86585	TB Tine Test	___
☐	87070	Culture	___
☐	70190	X-Ray; Optic Foramina	___
☐	70210	X-Ray Sinuses Complete	___
☐	71010	Radiological Exam Ent Spine	___
☐	71020	X-Ray Chest Pa & Lat	___
☐	72050	X-Ray Spine, Cerv (4 views)	___
☐	72090	X-Ray Spine; Scoliosis Ex	___
☐	72110	Spine, lumbosacral; a/p & Lat	___
☐	73030	Shoulder-Comp, min w/ 2vws	___
☐	73070	Elbow, anteropost & later vws	___
☐	73120	X-Ray; Hand, 2 views	___
☐	73560	X-Ray, Knee, 1 or 2 views	___
☐	74022	X-Ray; Abdomen, Complete	___
☐	75552	Cardiac Magnetic Res Img	___
☐	76020	X-Ray; Bone Age Studies	___
☐	77054	Mammary Ductogram Complete	___
☐	78465	Myocardial Perfusion Img	___

	CPT	DESCRIPTION	FEE
	PROCEDURES/TESTS		
☐	00452	Anesthesia for Rad Surgery	___
☐	11100	Skin Biopsy	___
☐	15852	Dressing Change	___
☐	29075	Cast Appl. - Lower Arm	___
☐	29530	Strapping of Knee	___
☐	29705	Removal/Revis of Cast w/Exa	___
☐	53670	Catheterization Incl. Suppl	___
☐	57452	Colposcopy	___
☐	57505	ECC	___
☐	69420	Myringotomy	___
☐	92081	Visual Field Examination	___
☐	92100	Serial Tonometry Exam	___
☐	92120	Tonography	___
☐	92552	Pure Tone Audiometry	___
☐	92567	Tympanometry	___
☐	93000	Electrocardiogram	___
☐	93015	Exercise Stress Test (ETT)	___
☐	93017	ETT Tracing Only	___
☐	93040	Electrocardiogram - Rhythm	___
☐	96100	Psychological Testing	___
☐	99000	Specimen Handling	___
☐	99058	Office Emergency Care	___
☐	99070	Surgical Tray - Misc.	___
☐	99080	Special Reports of Med Rec	___
☐	99195	Phlebotomy	___
☐	___	___	___
☐	___	___	___
☐	___	___	___

	ICD-9 CODE DIAGNOSIS
☐	009.0 Infect. colitis, enteritis, & gastroenteritis
☐	133.0 Scabies
☐	174.9 Breast Cancer, Female, Unspecified
☐	185 Malignant neoplasm of prostate
☐	250.00 Diabetes Mellitus w/o mention of Complication
☐	272.4 Hyperlipidemia
☐	282.5 Anemia, Sickle-cell Trait
☐	282.60 Sickle-cell disease, unspecified
☒	285.9 Anemia, Unspecified
☐	300.4 Dysthymic disorder
☐	340 Multiple Sclerosis
☐	342.90 Hemiplegia - Unspec.
☐	346.90 Migraine, unspecified
☐	352.9 Unspecified disorder of cranial nerves
☐	354.0 Carpal Tunnel Syndrome
☐	355.0 Sciatic Nerve Root Lesion
☐	366.9 Cataract
☐	386.00 Menier's disease, unspecified
☐	401.1 Essential Hypertension, Benign
☐	414.9 Ischemic Heart Disease
☐	428.0 Congestive Heart Failure (CHF), unspecified

	ICD-9 CODE DIAGNOSIS
☐	435.0 Basilar Artery Syndrome
☐	440.0 Atherosclerosis
☐	442.81 Carotid Artery
☐	460 Common Cold (Acute Nasopharyngitis)
☐	461.9 Acute Sinusitis
☐	474.00 Chronic Tonsillitis & Adenoiditis
☐	477.9 Allergic Rhinitis, Cause Unspecified
☐	487.0 Influenza with pneumonia
☐	496 Chronic Airway Obstruction
☐	522.0 Pulpitis
☐	524.60 Temporo-Mandibular Joint Disorder - Unspec.
☐	536.8 Stomach Pain
☐	553.3 Hiatal Hernia
☐	564.1 Spastic Colon
☐	574.40 Chronic Hepatitis, Unspecified
☐	571.5 Cirrhosis of Liver w/o mention of alcohol
☐	573.3 Hepatitis
☐	575.2 Obstruction of Gallbladder
☐	648.20 Anemia - Compl. Pregnancy
☐	715.90 Osteoarthritis - Unspec.
☐	721.3 Lumbar Osteo/Spondylarthrit

	ICD-9 CODE DIAGNOSIS
☐	724.2 Pain: Lower Back
☐	727.67 Rupture of Achilles Tendon
☐	780.1 Hallucinations
☐	780.3 Convulsions, Other
☐	780.50 Sleep Disturbances, Unspecified
☐	783.0 Anorexia
☐	783.1 Abnormal Weight Gain
☐	783.21 Abnormal Weight Loss
☐	823.80 Fractured Tibia
☐	823.81 Fractured Fibula
☐	831.00 Dislocated Shoulder, Closed, Unspecified
☐	835.00 Dislocated Hip, Closed, Unspecified
☐	842.00 Sprained Wrist, Unspecified Site
☐	845.00 Sprained Ankle, Unspecified Site
☐	919.5 Insect Bite, Nonvenomous
☐	921.1 Contus Eyelid/Perioc Area
☐	v16.3 Fam. Hist of Breast Cancer
☐	v17.4 Fam. Hist of Cardiovasc Dis
☐	v20.2 Well Child
☐	v22.0 Pregnancy - First Normal
☐	v22.1 Pregnancy - Normal

Previous Balance	Today's Charges	Total Due	Amount Paid	New Balance
___	___	___	___	___

Follow Up

PRN _____ Weeks _____ Months _____ Units _____

Next Appointment Date: _____   Time: _____

I hereby authorize release of any information acquired in the course of examination or treatment and allow a photocopy of my signature to be used.

_____

2. Based on the information found on the encounter form, enter the procedures and diagnosis for John Wyatt. After you have posted all the charges, compare your screen to Figure 3-6.

Figure 3-6 Three Posted Charges – Wyatt

```
Ṃ Student: Lois Fitzpatrick                                              _ 🗗 ✕
File  Edit  View  Windows  Help

🔲🕹🔲 🕐🔲🔲🔲 🔲🔲🔲 🔲🔲🔲🔲 🔲🔲🔲🔲                        🔲🔲 ✓🔲🔲

    Patient #: 307.0      [John Wyatt                     ]      Dept.   :  0
    Voucher #: 4032                Doctor #  :   1 Monroe MD, James   Location :
                                   Supervisor:   1 Monroe MD, James
    Dates     P.O.S.   Procedure   Modifier Diag. 1-4   Units      Charges   T.O.S.

    06/02/08   3        ▮.........                       .....   $    15.00  1

    |Blood Count, Manual Cell Count        |285.9      Anemia, Unspecified          |
    Comment:                               |                                        |
                                           |  .........                             |
                                           |  .........                             |
    Ins: Primary#: 6.0          Assign: Y   Secondary#: 0.0        EMC Billable: Y  |
    [Posted]
         Date       Co #  Dr# Procedure  Diag       Units      Charges  Total Chgs

      1  06/02/08 6     1   99213     285.9         1.00        40.00      40.00
      2  06/02/08 6     1   85014     285.9         1.00        18.00      58.00
      3  06/02/08 6     1   85032     285.9         1.00        15.00      73.00




        Enter '?', '!', '?code' for Help, '?~' for Macros, or '%' for Standing Orders



Ready                                                            NUM      🔲🔲🔲🔲
```

EXERCISE 4: MULTIPLE PROCEDURES WITH DIFFERENT DIAGNOSIS, MULTIPLE INSURANCE

CHRISTINE CUSACK

GOAL(S): In this exercise, you will need to match procedures with different diagnoses.

1. Before posting your entry, study the encounter form in Figure 3-7. Answer the following questions.

   a. What diagnosis would you match with the office visit? _____

   b. What diagnosis would you match with the cast application of the lower arm? _____

   c. How many procedures were completed at this visit? _____

   d. How many diagnoses are listed? _____

Figure 3-7   Encounter Form – Cusack

Sydney Carrington & Associates P.A.
34 Sycamore Street Suite 300
Madison, CA 95653

Date: 06/02/2008   Voucher No.: 4033

Time:

Patient: Christine Cusack   Patient No: 306.0
Guarantor: Doctor: 1 – J. Monroe

CPT	DESCRIPTION	FEE
OFFICE/HOSPITAL CONSULTS		
☐ 99201	Office New:Focused Hx-Exam	
☐ 99202	Office New:Expanded Hx.Exam	
☐ 99211	Office Estb:Min./None Hx-Exa	
☐ 99212	Office Estb:Focused Hx-Exam	
☐ 99213	Office Estb:Expanded Hx-Exa	
☒ 99214	Office Estb:Detailed Hx-Exa	
☐ 99215	Office Estb:Comprhn Hx-Exam	
☐ 99221	Hosp. Initial:Comprh Hx-	
☐ 99223	Hosp. Ini:Comprh Hx-Exam/Hi	
☐ 99231	Hosp. Subsequent: S-Fwd	
☐ 99232	Hosp. Subsequent: Comprhn Hx	
☐ 99233	Hosp. Subsequent: Ex/Hi	
☐ 99238	Hospital Visit Discharge Ex	
☐ 99371	Telephone Consult - Simple	
☐ 99372	Telephone Consult - Intermed	
☐ 99373	Telephone Consult - Complex	
☐ 90840	Counseling - 25 minutes	
☐ 90806	Counseling - 50 minutes	
☐ 90865	Counseling - Special Interview	
IMMUNIZATIONS/INJECTIONS		
☐ 90585	BCG Vaccine	
☐ 90659	Influenza Virus Vaccine	
☐ 90701	Immunization-DTP	
☐ 90702	DT Vaccine	
☐ 90703	Tetanus Toxoids	
☐ 90732	Pneumococcal Vaccine	
☐ 90746	Hepatitis B Vaccine	
☐ 90749	Immunization: Unlisted	

CPT	DESCRIPTION	FEE
LABORATORY/RADIOLOGY		
☐ 81000	Urinalysis	
☐ 81002	Urinalysis; Pregnancy Test	
☐ 82951	Glucose Tolerance Test	
☐ 84478	Triglycerides	
☐ 84550	Uric Acid: Blood Chemistry	
☐ 84830	Ovulation Test	
☐ 85014	Hematocrit	
☐ 85032	Hemogram, Complete Blood Wk	
☐ 86403	Particle Agglutination Test	
☐ 86485	Skin Test; Candida	
☐ 86580	TB Intradermal Test	
☐ 86585	TB Tine Test	
☐ 87070	Culture	
☐ 70190	X-Ray; Optic Foramina	
☐ 70210	X-Ray Sinuses Complete	
☐ 71010	Radiological Exam Ent Spine	
☐ 71020	X-Ray Chest Pa & Lat	
☐ 72050	X-Ray Spine, Cerv (4 views)	
☐ 72090	X-Ray Spine; Scoliosis Ex	
☐ 72110	Spine, lumbosacral; a/p & Lat	
☐ 73030	Shoulder-Comp, min w/ 2vws	
☐ 73070	Elbow, anteropost & later vws	
☐ 73120	X-Ray; Hand, 2 views	
☐ 73560	X-Ray, Knee, 1 or 2 views	
☐ 74022	X-Ray; Abdomen, Complete	
☐ 75552	Cardiac Magnetic Res Img	
☐ 76020	X-Ray; Bone Age Studies	
☐ 77054	Mammary Ductogram Complete	
☐ 78465	Myocardial Perfusion Img	

CPT	DESCRIPTION	FEE
PROCEDURES/TESTS		
☐ 00452	Anesthesia for Rad Surgery	
☐ 11100	Skin Biopsy	
☐ 15852	Dressing Change	
☒ 29075	Cast Appl. - Lower Arm	
☐ 29530	Strapping of Knee	
☐ 29705	Removal/Revis of Cast w/Exa	
☐ 53670	Catheterization Incl. Suppl	
☐ 57452	Colposcopy	
☐ 57505	ECC	
☐ 69420	Myringotomy	
☐ 92081	Visual Field Examination	
☐ 92100	Serial Tonometry Exam	
☐ 92120	Tonography	
☐ 92552	Pure Tone Audiometry	
☐ 92567	Tympanometry	
☐ 93000	Electrocardiogram	
☐ 93015	Exercise Stress Test (ETT)	
☐ 93017	ETT Tracing Only	
☐ 93040	Electrocardiogram - Rhythm	
☐ 96100	Psychological Testing	
☐ 99000	Specimen Handling	
☐ 99058	Office Emergency Care	
☐ 99070	Surgical Tray - Misc.	
☐ 99080	Special Reports of Med Rec	
☐ 99195	Phlebotomy	
☐		
☐		
☐		

ICD-9 CODE DIAGNOSIS	
☐ 009.0	Infect. colitis, enteritis, & gastroenteritis
☐ 133.0	Scabies
☐ 174.9	Breast Cancer, Female, Unspecified
☐ 185	Malignant neoplasm of prostate
☐ 250.00	Diabetes Mellitus w/o mention of Complication
☐ 272.4	Hyperlipidemia
☐ 282.5	Anemia, Sickle-cell Trait
☐ 282.60	Sickle-cell disease, unspecified
☐ 285.9	Anemia, Unspecified
☐ 300.4	Dysthymic disorder
☐ 340	Multiple Sclerosis
☐ 342.90	Hemiplegia - Unspec.
☐ 346.90	Migraine, unspecified
☐ 352.9	Unspecified disorder of cranial nerves
☐ 354.0	Carpal Tunnel Syndrome
☐ 355.0	Sciatic Nerve Root Lesion
☐ 366.9	Cataract
☐ 386.00	Menier's disease, unspecified
☐ 401.1	Essential Hypertension, Benign
☐ 414.9	Ischemic Heart Disease
☐ 428.0	Congestive Heart Failure (CHF), unspecified

ICD-9 CODE DIAGNOSIS	
☐ 435.0	Basilar Artery Syndrome
☐ 440.0	Atherosclerosis
☐ 442.81	Carotid Artery
☒ 460	Common Cold (Acute Nasopharyngitis)
☐ 461.9	Acute Sinusitis
☐ 474.00	Chronic Tonsillitis & Adenoiditis
☐ 477.9	Allergic Rhinitis, Cause Unspecified
☐ 487.0	Influenza with pneumonia
☐ 496	Chronic Airway Obstruction
☐ 522.0	Pulpitis
☐ 524.60	Temporo-Mandibular Joint Disorder - Unspec.
☐ 536.8	Stomach Pain
☐ 553.3	Hiatal Hernia
☐ 564.1	Spastic Colon
☐ 574.40	Chronic Hepatitis, Unspecified
☐ 571.5	Cirrhosis of Liver w/o mention of alcohol
☐ 573.3	Hepatitis
☐ 575.2	Obstruction of Gallbladder
☐ 648.20	Anemia - Compl. Pregnancy
☐ 715.90	Osteoarthritis - Unspec.
☐ 721.3	Lumbar Osteo/Spondylarthrit

ICD-9 CODE DIAGNOSIS	
☐ 724.2	Pain: Lower Back
☐ 727.67	Rupture of Achilles Tendon
☐ 780.1	Hallucinations
☐ 780.3	Convulsions, Other
☐ 780.50	Sleep Disturbances, Unspecified
☐ 783.0	Anorexia
☐ 783.1	Abnormal Weight Gain
☐ 783.21	Abnormal Weight Loss
☐ 823.80	Fractured Tibia
☐ 823.81	Fractured Fibula
☐ 831.00	Dislocated Shoulder, Closed, Unspecified
☐ 835.00	Dislocated Hip, Closed, Unspecified
☒ 842.00	Sprained Wrist, Unspecified Site
☐ 845.00	Sprained Ankle, Unspecified Site
☐ 919.5	Insect Bite, Nonvenomous
☐ 921.1	Contus Eyelid/Perioc Area
☐ v16.3	Fam. Hist of Breast Cancer
☐ v17.4	Fam. Hist of Cardiovasc Dis
☐ v20.2	Well Child
☐ v22.0	Pregnancy - First Normal
☐ v22.1	Pregnancy - Normal

Previous Balance	Today's Charges	Total Due	Amount Paid	New Balance

Follow Up

PRN _____ Weeks _____ Months _____ Units _____

Next Appointment Date: _____   Time: _____

I hereby authorize release of any information acquired in the course of examination or treatment and allow a photocopy of my signature to be used.

2. Based on the information found on the encounter form, enter the procedures and diagnoses for Christine Cusack. After posting both charges, compare your screen to Figure 3-8.

Figure 3-8   Two Procedures Posted – Cusack

```
M Student: Lois Fitzpatrick                                                    _ □ ✕
File  Edit  View  Windows  Help

 ▒▓ ▒ ▒ ▒ ▒ ▒ ▒ ▒  ▒▒▒▒  ▒▒▒▒  ▒▒▒                              ▒▒ ▒ ✓ ? ▒

   Patient #: 306.0     [Christine Cusack          ]       Dept.  :  0
   Voucher #: 4033               Doctor # :  1 Monroe MD, James   Location :
                                 Supervisor:  1 Monroe MD, James
   Dates    P.O.S.  Procedure   Modifier Diag. 1-4    Units      Charges  T.O.S.

   06/02/08  3       ..........                       .....   $    48.00  1

   |Cast Application, Elbow to Finger  |842.00    Sprained Wrist, Unspecified Si|
   Comment:                           |
                                      |    ..........
                                      |    ..........
   Ins: Primary#: 7.1        Assign: Y     Secondary#: 5.0       EMC Billable: Y
   [Posted]───────────────────────────────────────────────────────────────────
        Date      Co #  Dr# Procedure   Diag      Units     Charges   Total Chgs

    1  06/02/08  7    1   99214      460          1.00      50.00       50.00
    2  06/02/08  7    1   29075      842.00       1.00      48.00       98.00




        Enter '?', '!', '?code' for Help, '?~' for Macros, or '%' for Standing Orders



 Ready                                                              NUM   ↑↓⟵⟶
```

EXERCISE 5: MULTIPLE PROCEDURES, ONE DIAGNOSIS, ONE INSURANCE FOR PATIENT WITH DIFFERENT LAST NAME

MATTHEW NOONAN

GOAL(S): In this exercise, you will enter procedures and a diagnosis for a patient with a last name different from the guarantor.

1. Before posting your entry, study the encounter form in Figure 3-9. Answer the following questions.

   a. Who is the patient? _____

   b. How will you need to search for this patient who has a last name different from the guarantor?

   _____

   c. How many procedures were completed at this visit? _____

   d. How many diagnoses are listed? _____

Figure 3-9 Encounter Form – Noonan

Sydney Carrington & Associates P.A.
34 Sycamore Street Suite 300
Madison, CA 95653

Date: 06/02/2008

Voucher No.: 4034

Time:

Patient: Matthew Noonan
Guarantor:

Patient No: 310.1
Doctor: 2 – F. Simpson

□	CPT	DESCRIPTION	FEE
		OFFICE/HOSPITAL CONSULTS	
□	99201	Office New:Focused Hx-Exam	
□	99202	Office New:Expanded Hx.Exam	
□	99211	Office Estb:Min./None Hx-Exa	
□	99212	Office Estb:Focused Hx-Exam	
☒	99213	Office Estb:Expanded Hx-Exa	
□	99214	Office Estb:Detailed Hx-Exa	
□	99215	Office Estb:Comprhn Hx-Exam	
□	99221	Hosp. Initial:Comprh Hx-	
□	99223	Hosp. Ini:Comprh Hx-Exam/Hi	
□	99231	Hosp. Subsequent: S-Fwd	
□	99232	Hosp. Subsequent: Comprhn Hx	
□	99233	Hosp. Subsequent: Ex/Hi	
□	99238	Hospital Visit Discharge Ex	
□	99371	Telephone Consult - Simple	
□	99372	Telephone Consult - Intermed	
□	99373	Telephone Consult - Complex	
□	90840	Counseling - 25 minutes	
☒	90806	Counseling - 50 minutes	
□	90865	Counseling - Special Interview	
		IMMUNIZATIONS/INJECTIONS	
□	90585	BCG Vaccine	
□	90659	Influenza Virus Vaccine	
□	90701	Immunization-DTP	
□	90702	DT Vaccine	
□	90703	Tetanus Toxoids	
□	90732	Pneumococcal Vaccine	
□	90746	Hepatitis B Vaccine	
□	90749	Immunization: Unlisted	

□	CPT	DESCRIPTION	FEE
		LABORATORY/RADIOLOGY	
□	81000	Urinalysis	
□	81002	Urinalysis; Pregnancy Test	
□	82951	Glucose Tolerance Test	
□	84478	Triglycerides	
□	84550	Uric Acid: Blood Chemistry	
□	84830	Ovulation Test	
□	85014	Hematocrit	
□	85032	Hemogram, Complete Blood Wk	
□	86403	Particle Agglutination Test	
□	86485	Skin Test; Candida	
□	86580	TB Intradermal Test	
□	86585	TB Tine Test	
□	87070	Culture	
□	70190	X-Ray; Optic Foramina	
□	70210	X-Ray Sinuses Complete	
□	71010	Radiological Exam Ent Spine	
□	71020	X-Ray Chest Pa & Lat	
□	72050	X-Ray Spine, Cerv (4 views)	
□	72090	X-Ray Spine; Scoliosis Ex	
□	72110	Spine, lumbosacral; a/p & Lat	
□	73030	Shoulder-Comp, min w/ 2vws	
□	73070	Elbow, anteropost & later vws	
□	73120	X-Ray; Hand, 2 views	
□	73560	X-Ray, Knee, 1 or 2 views	
□	74022	X-Ray; Abdomen, Complete	
□	75552	Cardiac Magnetic Res Img	
□	76020	X-Ray; Bone Age Studies	
□	77054	Mammary Ductogram Complete	
□	78465	Myocardial Perfusion Img	

□	CPT	DESCRIPTION	FEE
		PROCEDURES/TESTS	
□	00452	Anesthesia for Rad Surgery	
□	11100	Skin Biopsy	
□	15852	Dressing Change	
□	29075	Cast Appl. - Lower Arm	
□	29530	Strapping of Knee	
□	29705	Removal/Revis of Cast w/Exa	
□	53670	Catheterization Incl. Suppl	
□	57452	Colposcopy	
□	57505	ECC	
□	69420	Myringotomy	
□	92081	Visual Field Examination	
□	92100	Serial Tonometry Exam	
□	92120	Tonography	
□	92552	Pure Tone Audiometry	
□	92567	Tympanometry	
□	93000	Electrocardiogram	
□	93015	Exercise Stress Test (ETT)	
□	93017	ETT Tracing Only	
□	93040	Electrocardiogram - Rhythm	
□	96100	Psychological Testing	
□	99000	Specimen Handling	
□	99058	Office Emergency Care	
□	99070	Surgical Tray - Misc.	
□	99080	Special Reports of Med Rec	
□	99195	Phlebotomy	
□			
□			
□			
□			

□	ICD-9 CODE DIAGNOSIS	
□	009.0	Infect. colitis, enteritis, & gastroenteritis
□	133.0	Scabies
□	174.9	Breast Cancer, Female, Unspecified
□	185	Malignant neoplasm of prostate
□	250.00	Diabetes Mellitus w/o mention of Complication
□	272.4	Hyperlipidemia
□	282.5	Anemia, Sickle-cell Trait
□	282.60	Sickle-cell disease, unspecified
□	285.9	Anemia, Unspecified
□	300.4	Dysthymic disorder
□	340	Multiple Sclerosis
□	342.90	Hemiplegia - Unspec.
□	346.90	Migraine, unspecified
□	352.9	Unspecified disorder of cranial nerves
□	354.0	Carpal Tunnel Syndrome
□	355.0	Sciatic Nerve Root Lesion
□	366.9	Cataract
□	386.00	Menier's disease, unspecified
□	401.1	Essential Hypertension, Benign
□	414.9	Ischemic Heart Disease
□	428.0	Congestive Heart Failure (CHF), unspecified

□	ICD-9 CODE DIAGNOSIS	
□	435.0	Basilar Artery Syndrome
□	440.0	Atherosclerosis
□	442.81	Carotid Artery
□	460	Common Cold (Acute Nasopharyngitis)
□	461.9	Acute Sinusitis
□	474.00	Chronic Tonsillitis & Adenoiditis
□	477.9	Allergic Rhinitis, Cause Unspecified
□	487.0	Influenza with pneumonia
□	496	Chronic Airway Obstruction
□	522.0	Pulpitis
□	524.60	Temporo-Mandibular Joint Disorder - Unspec.
□	536.8	Stomach Pain
□	553.3	Hiatal Hernia
□	564.1	Spastic Colon
□	574.40	Chronic Hepatitis, Unspecified
□	571.5	Cirrhosis of Liver w/o mention of alcohol
□	573.3	Hepatitis
□	575.2	Obstruction of Gallbladder
□	648.20	Anemia - Compl. Pregnancy
□	715.90	Osteoarthritis - Unspec.
□	721.3	Lumbar Osteo/Spondylarthrit

□	ICD-9 CODE DIAGNOSIS	
□	724.2	Pain: Lower Back
□	727.67	Rupture of Achilles Tendon
□	780.1	Hallucinations
□	780.3	Convulsions, Other
☒	780.50	Sleep Disturbances, Unspecified
□	783.0	Anorexia
□	783.1	Abnormal Weight Gain
□	783.21	Abnormal Weight Loss
□	823.80	Fractured Tibia
□	823.81	Fractured Fibula
□	831.00	Dislocated Shoulder, Closed, Unspecified
□	835.00	Dislocated Hip, Closed, Unspecified
□	842.00	Sprained Wrist, Unspecified Site
□	845.00	Sprained Ankle, Unspecified Site
□	919.5	Insect Bite, Nonvenomous
□	921.1	Contus Eyelid/Perioc Area
□	v16.3	Fam. Hist of Breast Cancer
□	v17.4	Fam. Hist of Cardiovasc Dis
□	v20.2	Well Child
□	v22.0	Pregnancy - First Normal
□	v22.1	Pregnancy - Normal

Previous Balance	Today's Charges	Total Due	Amount Paid	New Balance

Follow Up

PRN _____ Weeks _____ Months _____ Units _____

Next Appointment Date: _____   Time: _____

I hereby authorize release of any information acquired in the course of examination or treatment and allow a photocopy of my signature to be used.

_____

2. Based on the information found on the encounter form, enter the procedures and diagnoses for Matthew Noonan. After posting the procedures, compare your screen to Figure 3-10.

Figure 3-10 Two Procedures Posted – Noonan

```
M Student: Lois Fitzpatrick                                                    _ |□|X|
File  Edit  View  Windows  Help
╔═╗ ╔═╗ ... toolbar icons ...                                          ... ✓ ? ...

  Patient #:  310.1      [Matthew Noonan              ]      Dept.   :  0
  Voucher #:  4034              Doctor #  :   2 Simpson M.D., Fran  Location :
                                Supervisor:   2 Simpson M.D., Fran
  Dates    P.O.S.   Procedure   Modifier Diag. 1-4   Units      Charges   T.O.S.
  ─────────────────────────────────────────────────────────────────────────
  06/02/08   3      ..........                         .....  $    120.00  1

  |Counseling - 45 - 50 Minutes, Face |780.50     Sleep Disturbances, Unspecifie|
  Comment:                            |
                                      |        ..........
                                      |        ..........
  Ins: Primary#: 5.0         Assign: Y    Secondary#: 0.0       EMC Billable: Y
  [Posted]─────────────────────────────────────────────────────────────────
        Date       Co #   Dr# Procedure   Diag      Units     Charges   Total Chgs

    1   06/02/08  5     2    99213      780.50       1.00      40.00       40.00
    2   06/02/08  5     2    90806      780.50       1.00     120.00      160.00




     Enter '?', '!', '?code' for Help, '?~' for Macros, or '%' for Standing Orders



Ready                                                              NUM    ↑↓⇐⇒
```

EXERCISE 6: WORKER'S COMPENSATION WITH AILMENT

ROBERTO VEGA

GOAL(S): In this exercise, you will enter procedures and a diagnosis for a patient who was injured at work. This is a worker's compensation case, therefore, you will need to add Ailment Detail for the insurance company.

1. Before posting your entry, study the encounter form in Figure 3-11. Answer the following questions.

   a. Who is the patient? _____

   b. How many procedures were completed at this visit? _____

   c. After adding the Ailment Detail for the first procedure, what response to Ailment Detail is entered for the remaining procedures? _____

   d. How many diagnoses are listed? _____

Figure 3-11   Encounter Form – Vega

Sydney Carrington & Associates P.A.
34 Sycamore Street Suite 300
Madison, CA 95653

Date: 06/02/2008   Voucher No.: 4035

Time:

Patient: Roberto Vega   Patient No: 311.1
Guarantor: Doctor: 1 - J. Monroe

☐	CPT	DESCRIPTION	FEE
	OFFICE/HOSPITAL CONSULTS		
☐	99201	Office New:Focused Hx-Exam	___
☐	99202	Office New:Expanded Hx.Exam	___
☐	99211	Office Estb:Min./None Hx-Exa	___
☐	99212	Office Estb:Focused Hx-Exam	___
☐	99213	Office Estb:Expanded Hx-Exa	___
☒	99214	Office Estb:Detailed Hx-Exa	___
☐	99215	Office Estb:Comprhn Hx-Exam	___
☐	99221	Hosp. Initial:Comprh Hx-	___
☐	99223	Hosp. Ini:Comprh Hx-Exam/Hi	___
☐	99231	Hosp. Subsequent: S-Fwd	___
☐	99232	Hosp. Subsequent: Comprhn Hx	___
☐	99233	Hosp. Subsequent: Ex/Hi	___
☐	99238	Hospital Visit Discharge Ex	___
☐	99371	Telephone Consult - Simple	___
☐	99372	Telephone Consult - Intermed	___
☐	99373	Telephone Consult - Complex	___
☐	90840	Counseling - 25 minutes	___
☐	90806	Counseling - 50 minutes	___
☐	90865	Counseling - Special Interview	___
	IMMUNIZATIONS/INJECTIONS		
☐	90585	BCG Vaccine	___
☐	90659	Influenza Virus Vaccine	___
☐	90701	Immunization-DTP	___
☐	90702	DT Vaccine	___
☐	90703	Tetanus Toxoids	___
☐	90732	Pneumococcal Vaccine	___
☐	90746	Hepatitis B Vaccine	___
☐	90749	Immunization: Unlisted	___

☐	CPT	DESCRIPTION	FEE
	LABORATORY/RADIOLOGY		
☐	81000	Urinalysis	___
☐	81002	Urinalysis; Pregnancy Test	___
☐	82951	Glucose Tolerance Test	___
☐	84478	Triglycerides	___
☐	84550	Uric Acid: Blood Chemistry	___
☐	84830	Ovulation Test	___
☐	85014	Hematocrit	___
☐	85032	Hemogram, Complete Blood Wk	___
☐	86403	Particle Agglutination Test	___
☐	86485	Skin Test; Candida	___
☐	86580	TB Intradermal Test	___
☐	86585	TB Tine Test	___
☐	87070	Culture	___
☐	70190	X-Ray; Optic Foramina	___
☐	70210	X-Ray Sinuses Complete	___
☐	71010	Radiological Exam Ent Spine	___
☐	71020	X-Ray Chest Pa & Lat	___
☒	72050	X-Ray Spine, Cerv (4 views)	___
☐	72090	X-Ray Spine; Scoliosis Ex	___
☐	72110	Spine, lumbosacral; a/p & Lat	___
☐	73030	Shoulder-Comp, min w/ 2vws	___
☐	73070	Elbow, anteropost & later vws	___
☐	73120	X-Ray; Hand, 2 views	___
☐	73560	X-Ray; Knee, 1 or 2 views	___
☐	74022	X-Ray; Abdomen, Complete	___
☐	75552	Cardiac Magnetic Res Img	___
☐	76020	X-Ray; Bone Age Studies	___
☐	77054	Mammary Ductogram Complete	___
☐	78465	Myocardial Perfusion Img	___

☐	CPT	DESCRIPTION	FEE
	PROCEDURES/TESTS		
☐	00452	Anesthesia for Rad Surgery	___
☐	11100	Skin Biopsy	___
☐	15852	Dressing Change	___
☐	29075	Cast Appl. - Lower Arm	___
☐	29530	Strapping of Knee	___
☐	29705	Removal/Revis of Cast w/Exa	___
☐	53670	Catheterization Incl. Suppl	___
☐	57452	Colposcopy	___
☐	57505	ECC	___
☐	69420	Myringotomy	___
☐	92081	Visual Field Examination	___
☐	92100	Serial Tonometry Exam	___
☐	92120	Tonography	___
☐	92552	Pure Tone Audiometry	___
☐	92567	Tympanometry	___
☐	93000	Electrocardiogram	___
☐	93015	Exercise Stress Test (ETT)	___
☐	93017	ETT Tracing Only	___
☐	93040	Electrocardiogram - Rhythm	___
☐	96100	Psychological Testing	___
☐	99000	Specimen Handling	___
☐	99058	Office Emergency Care	___
☐	99070	Surgical Tray - Misc.	___
☐	99080	Special Reports of Med Rec	___
☐	99195	Phlebotomy	___
☐		_____	___
☐		_____	___
☐		_____	___

☐	**ICD-9 CODE DIAGNOSIS**
☐ 009.0	Infect. colitis, enteritis, & gastroenteritis
☐ 133.0	Scabies
☐ 174.9	Breast Cancer, Female, Unspecified
☐ 185	Malignant neoplasm of prostate
☐ 250.00	Diabetes Mellitus w/o mention of Complication
☐ 272.4	Hyperlipidemia
☐ 282.5	Anemia, Sickle-cell Trait
☐ 282.60	Sickle-cell disease, unspecified
☐ 285.9	Anemia, Unspecified
☐ 300.4	Dysthymic disorder
☐ 340	Multiple Sclerosis
☐ 342.90	Hemiplegia - Unspec.
☐ 346.90	Migraine, unspecified
☐ 352.9	Unspecified disorder of cranial nerves
☐ 354.0	Carpal Tunnel Syndrome
☐ 355.0	Sciatic Nerve Root Lesion
☐ 366.9	Cataract
☐ 386.00	Menier's disease, unspecified
☐ 401.1	Essential Hypertension, Benign
☐ 414.9	Ischemic Heart Disease
☐ 428.0	Congestive Heart Failure (CHF), unspecified

☐	**ICD-9 CODE DIAGNOSIS**
☐ 435.0	Basilar Artery Syndrome
☐ 440.0	Atherosclerosis
☐ 442.81	Carotid Artery
☐ 460	Common Cold (Acute Nasopharyngitis)
☐ 461.9	Acute Sinusitis
☐ 474.00	Chronic Tonsillitis & Adenoiditis
☐ 477.9	Allergic Rhinitis, Cause Unspecified
☐ 487.0	Influenza with pneumonia
☐ 496	Chronic Airway Obstruction
☐ 522.0	Pulpitis
☐ 524.60	Temporo-Mandibular Joint Disorder - Unspec.
☐ 536.8	Stomach Pain
☐ 553.3	Hiatal Hernia
☐ 564.1	Spastic Colon
☐ 574.40	Chronic Hepatitis, Unspecified
☐ 571.5	Cirrhosis of Liver w/o mention of alcohol
☐ 573.3	Hepatitis
☐ 575.2	Obstruction of Gallbladder
☐ 648.20	Anemia - Compl. Pregnancy
☐ 715.90	Osteoarthritis - Unspec.
☐ 721.3	Lumbar Osteo/Spondylarthrit

☐	**ICD-9 CODE DIAGNOSIS**
☒ 724.2	Pain: Lower Back
☐ 727.67	Rupture of Achilles Tendon
☐ 780.1	Hallucinations
☐ 780.3	Convulsions, Other
☐ 780.50	Sleep Disturbances, Unspecified
☐ 783.0	Anorexia
☐ 783.1	Abnormal Weight Gain
☐ 783.21	Abnormal Weight Loss
☐ 823.80	Fractured Tibia
☐ 823.81	Fractured Fibula
☐ 831.00	Dislocated Shoulder, Closed, Unspecified
☐ 835.00	Dislocated Hip, Closed, Unspecified
☐ 842.00	Sprained Wrist, Unspecified Site
☐ 845.00	Sprained Ankle, Unspecified Site
☐ 919.5	Insect Bite, Nonvenomous
☐ 921.1	Contus Eyelid/Perioc Area
☐ v16.3	Fam. Hist of Breast Cancer
☐ v17.4	Fam. Hist of Cardiovasc Dis
☐ v20.2	Well Child
☐ v22.0	Pregnancy - First Normal
☐ v22.1	Pregnancy - Normal

Previous Balance	Today's Charges	Total Due	Amount Paid	New Balance
_____	_____	_____	_____	_____

Follow Up

PRN _____ Weeks _____ Months _____ Units _____

Next Appointment Date: Time:

I hereby authorize release of any information acquired in the course of examination or treatment and allow a photocopy of my signature to be used.

_____

2. Based on the information found on the encounter form, enter the procedures and diagnosis for Roberto Vega. When prompted for Ailment Detail, use the following information to complete the Ailment Detail screen (accept default response if not indicated):

Hold Claim: (N)ormal Billing

Date First Consulted: 06/02/2008

Comment Field: WC Back

Related to Employment: (Y)es

Accident: (O)ther

Old Symptom: (N)o

Emergency: (N)o

Date of first symptom: 06/02/2008

Date last worked: 06/02/2008

Date resumed work: 06/03/2008

Dates of Disability : 06/02/2008 to (LEAVE BLANK)

Disability: (S)hort Term

Compare your screens to Figures 3-12 and 3-13.

Figure 3-12 Ailment Detail – Vega

```
M Student: Lois Fitzpatrick                                          _ □ X
File  Edit  View  Windows  Help
 ⊞ ⋮ ⋮ | ⊙ ⋮ ⋮ ⋮ | /S ⋮ ⋮ | ⊞ ⊞ ⋮ ⋮ | ⋮ ⋮ ⋮ ⋮           ⬚ ⬚  ✓ ? ⬚

    Patient : Vega, Roberto                          Use Cnt : 1
    Hold Claim (Y/N/I): N             Comment Field : WC Back    Inpatient: N
    Date 1st Consulted: 06/02/08          Specialty:
    Facility #:     [                ]
    Authorization 1:                      Auth 1 Type :    Ins 1 :
    Authorization 2:                      Auth 2 Type :    Ins 2 :


    Ref Dr : 3     [Lucinda A Fredericks M.D.      ]
    Related to Employment (Y/N)     : Y       Old Symptom (Y/N)    : N
    ACCIDENT:(A)uto,(O)ther,(N)one  : O       Emergency (Y/N)      : N


    Date 1st Symptom  : 06/02/08   Special         :
    Date Last Worked  : 06/02/08   Date Resumed Work : 06/03/08


    Dates of Disability       : 06/02/08 to           Disability : S Short
    Dates of Similar Illness  :          to
    Dates of Hospitalization  :          to
    Dates Assume/Relinquish Care :       to


    Outside Lab (Y/N)   :             EPSDT           (Y/N)  :
    Lab Charges         :    0.00     Family Planning (Y/N)  :
    Lab Facility #      :    [                ] Delay Reason :

     Enter 'Y' to Postpone Insurance Billing, 'N' for Normal, or 'I' for Instant


Ready                                                        NUM    ↑↓◄►
```

Figure 3-13 Two Procedures Posted – Vega

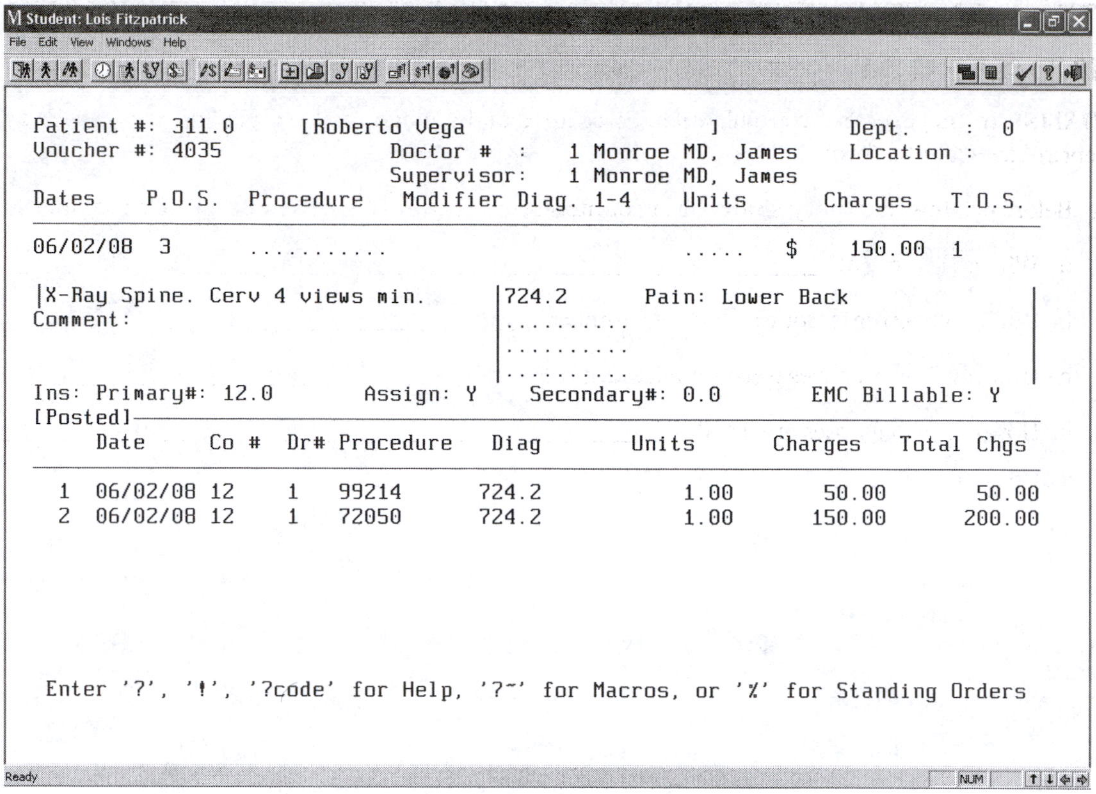

```
Ⅶ Student: Lois Fitzpatrick                                                    _ ⬚ ✕
File  Edit  View  Windows  Help

  Patient #: 311.0     [Roberto Vega                  ]     Dept.    : 0
  Voucher #: 4035               Doctor #  :  1 Monroe MD, James  Location :
                                Supervisor:  1 Monroe MD, James
  Dates    P.O.S.  Procedure   Modifier Diag. 1-4    Units      Charges   T.O.S.
  ─────────────────────────────────────────────────────────────────────────
  06/02/08  3        ..........                        .....   $  150.00  1

  |X-Ray Spine. Cerv 4 views min.     |724.2      Pain: Lower Back
  Comment:                            |   ..........
                                      |   ..........
                                      |   ..........
  Ins: Primary#: 12.0       Assign: Y    Secondary#: 0.0      EMC Billable: Y
  [Posted]────────────────────────────────────────────────────────────────
        Date    Co #  Dr# Procedure    Diag        Units       Charges  Total Chgs
  ─────────────────────────────────────────────────────────────────────────
     1  06/02/08 12    1   99214       724.2        1.00        50.00     50.00
     2  06/02/08 12    1   72050       724.2        1.00       150.00    200.00




     Enter '?', '!', '?code' for Help, '?~' for Macros, or '%' for Standing Orders


Ready                                                              NUM    ↑↓◄►
```

EXERCISE 7: WORK-INS

LINDA FROST

GOAL(S): In this exercise, you will enter procedures and a diagnosis for a patient who does not have a preprinted encounter form.

 1. Before posting your entry, study the encounter form in Figure 3-14. Answer the following questions.

 a. Who is the patient? _____

 b. What will you enter for the voucher number? _____

 c. How many procedures were completed at this visit? _____

 d. How many diagnoses are listed? _____

Figure 3-14   Encounter Form – Frost

Sydney Carrington & Associates P.A.
34 Sycamore Street Suite 300
Madison, CA 95653

Date: 06/02/2008   Voucher No.: Work-In

Time:

Patient: Linda Frost   Patient No: 308.1
Guarantor: Doctor: 3 – S. Carrington

☐ CPT	DESCRIPTION	FEE	☐ CPT	DESCRIPTION	FEE	☐ CPT	DESCRIPTION	FEE
OFFICE/HOSPITAL CONSULTS			**LABORATORY/RADIOLOGY**			**PROCEDURES/TESTS**		
☐ 99201	Office New:Focused Hx-Exam		☐ 81000	Urinalysis		☐ 00452	Anesthesia for Rad Surgery	
☐ 99202	Office New:Expanded Hx.Exam		☐ 81002	Urinalysis; Pregnancy Test		☐ 11100	Skin Biopsy	
☐ 99211	Office Estb:Min./None Hx-Exa		☐ 82951	Glucose Tolerance Test		☐ 15852	Dressing Change	
☐ 99212	Office Estb:Focused Hx-Exam		☐ 84478	Triglycerides		☐ 29075	Cast Appl. - Lower Arm	
☒ 99213	Office Estb:Expanded Hx-Exa		☐ 84550	Uric Acid: Blood Chemistry		☐ 29530	Strapping of Knee	
☐ 99214	Office Estb:Detailed Hx-Exa		☐ 84830	Ovulation Test		☐ 29705	Removal/Revis of Cast w/Exa	
☐ 99215	Office Estb:Comprhn Hx-Exam		☐ 85014	Hematocrit		☐ 53670	Catheterization Incl. Suppl	
☐ 99221	Hosp. Initial:Comprh Hx-		☐ 85032	Hemogram, Complete Blood Wk		☐ 57452	Colposcopy	
☐ 99223	Hosp. Ini:Comprh Hx-Exam/Hi		☐ 86403	Particle Agglutination Test		☐ 57505	ECC	
☐ 99231	Hosp. Subsequent: S-Fwd		☐ 86485	Skin Test; Candida		☐ 69420	Myringotomy	
☐ 99232	Hosp. Subsequent: Comprhn Hx		☐ 86580	TB Intradermal Test		☐ 92081	Visual Field Examination	
☐ 99233	Hosp. Subsequent: Ex/Hi		☐ 86585	TB Tine Test		☐ 92100	Serial Tonometry Exam	
☐ 99238	Hospital Visit Discharge Ex		☒ 87070	Culture		☐ 92120	Tonography	
☐ 99371	Telephone Consult - Simple		☐ 70190	X-Ray; Optic Foramina		☐ 92552	Pure Tone Audiometry	
☐ 99372	Telephone Consult - Intermed		☐ 70210	X-Ray Sinuses Complete		☐ 92567	Tympanometry	
☐ 99373	Telephone Consult - Complex		☐ 71010	Radiological Exam Ent Spine		☐ 93000	Electrocardiogram	
☐ 90840	Counseling - 25 minutes		☐ 71020	X-Ray Chest Pa & Lat		☐ 93015	Exercise Stress Test (ETT)	
☐ 90806	Counseling - 50 minutes		☐ 72050	X-Ray Spine, Cerv (4 views)		☐ 93017	ETT Tracing Only	
☐ 90865	Counseling - Special Interview		☐ 72090	X-Ray Spine; Scoliosis Ex		☐ 93040	Electrocardiogram - Rhythm	
			☐ 72110	Spine, lumbosacral; a/p & Lat		☐ 96100	Psychological Testing	
IMMUNIZATIONS/INJECTIONS			☐ 73030	Shoulder-Comp, min w/ 2vws		☐ 99000	Specimen Handling	
☐ 90585	BCG Vaccine		☐ 73070	Elbow, anteropost & later vws		☐ 99058	Office Emergency Care	
☐ 90659	Influenza Virus Vaccine		☐ 73120	X-Ray; Hand, 2 views		☐ 99070	Surgical Tray - Misc.	
☐ 90701	Immunization-DTP		☐ 73560	X-Ray, Knee, 1 or 2 views		☐ 99080	Special Reports of Med Rec	
☐ 90702	DT Vaccine		☐ 74022	X-Ray; Abdomen, Complete		☐ 99195	Phlebotomy	
☐ 90703	Tetanus Toxoids		☐ 75552	Cardiac Magnetic Res Img		☐		
☐ 90732	Pneumococcal Vaccine		☐ 76020	X-Ray; Bone Age Studies		☐		
☐ 90746	Hepatitis B Vaccine		☐ 77054	Mammary Ductogram Complete		☐		
☐ 90749	Immunization: Unlisted		☐ 78465	Myocardial Perfusion Img		☐		

☐ ICD-9 CODE DIAGNOSIS		☐ ICD-9 CODE DIAGNOSIS		☐ ICD-9 CODE DIAGNOSIS	
☐ 009.0	Infect. colitis, enteritis, & gastroenteritis	☐ 435.0	Basilar Artery Syndrome	☒ 724.2	Pain: Lower Back
☐ 133.0	Scabies	☐ 440.0	Atherosclerosis	☐ 727.67	Rupture of Achilles Tendon
☐ 174.9	Breast Cancer, Female, Unspecified	☐ 442.81	Carotid Artery	☐ 780.1	Hallucinations
☐ 185	Malignant neoplasm of prostate	☐ 460	Common Cold (Acute Nasopharyngitis)	☐ 780.3	Convulsions, Other
☐ 250.00	Diabetes Mellitus w/o mention of Complication	☐ 461.9	Acute Sinusitis	☐ 780.50	Sleep Disturbances, Unspecified
☐ 272.4	Hyperlipidemia	☒ 474.00	Chronic Tonsillitis & Adenoiditis	☐ 783.0	Anorexia
☐ 282.5	Anemia, Sickle-cell Trait	☐ 477.9	Allergic Rhinitis, Cause Unspecified	☐ 783.1	Abnormal Weight Gain
☐ 282.60	Sickle-cell disease, unspecified	☐ 487.0	Influenza with pneumonia	☐ 783.21	Abnormal Weight Loss
☐ 285.9	Anemia, Unspecified	☐ 496	Chronic Airway Obstruction	☐ 823.80	Fractured Tibia
☐ 300.4	Dysthymic disorder	☐ 522.0	Pulpitis	☐ 823.81	Fractured Fibula
☐ 340	Multiple Sclerosis	☐ 524.60	Temporo-Mandibular Joint Disorder - Unspec.	☐ 831.00	Dislocated Shoulder, Closed, Unspecified
☐ 342.90	Hemiplegia - Unspec.	☐ 536.8	Stomach Pain	☐ 835.00	Dislocated Hip, Closed, Unspecified
☐ 346.90	Migraine, unspecified	☐ 553.3	Hiatal Hernia	☐ 842.00	Sprained Wrist, Unspecified Site
☐ 352.9	Unspecified disorder of cranial nerves	☐ 564.1	Spastic Colon	☐ 845.00	Sprained Ankle, Unspecified Site
☐ 354.0	Carpal Tunnel Syndrome	☐ 574.40	Chronic Hepatitis, Unspecified	☐ 919.5	Insect Bite, Nonvenomous
☐ 355.0	Sciatic Nerve Root Lesion	☐ 571.5	Cirrhosis of Liver w/o mention of alcohol	☐ 921.1	Contus Eyelid/Perioc Area
☐ 366.9	Cataract	☐ 573.3	Hepatitis	☐ v16.3	Fam. Hist of Breast Cancer
☐ 386.00	Menier's disease, unspecified	☐ 575.2	Obstruction of Gallbladder	☐ v17.4	Fam. Hist of Cardiovasc Dis
☐ 401.1	Essential Hypertension, Benign	☐ 648.20	Anemia - Compl. Pregnancy	☐ v20.2	Well Child
☐ 414.9	Ischemic Heart Disease	☐ 715.90	Osteoarthritis - Unspec.	☐ v22.0	Pregnancy - First Normal
☐ 428.0	Congestive Heart Failure (CHF), unspecified	☐ 721.3	Lumbar Osteo/Spondylarthrit	☐ v22.1	Pregnancy - Normal

Previous Balance	Today's Charges	Total Due	Amount Paid	New Balance		Follow Up
_____	_____	_____	_____	_____	PRN _____ Weeks _____	Months _____ Units _____
					Next Appointment Date:	Time:

I hereby authorize release of any information acquired in the course of
examination or treatment and allow a photocopy of my signature to be used.

_____   _____

2. Based on the information found on the encounter form, enter the procedures and diagnosis for Linda Frost. After posting all charges, compare your screen to Figure 3-15.

Figure 3-15   Two Procedures Posted – Frost

```
 Student: Lois Fitzpatrick                                                    _ □ X
File  Edit  View  Windows  Help

Patient #: 308.1      [Linda Frost                    ]      Dept.    :   0
Voucher #: WorkIn              Doctor #  :   3 Carrington M.D., S  Location :
                               Supervisor:  3 Carrington M.D., S
Dates     P.O.S.   Procedure   Modifier Diag. 1-4    Units       Charges   T.O.S.

06/02/08   3        ■.........                        .....  $      31.00   1

|Culture                              |474.00      Chronic Tonsillitis & Adenoidi|
Comment:                              |
                                      |..........
                                      |..........
Ins: Primary#: 11.0        Assign: Y    Secondary#: 0.0       EMC Billable: Y
[Posted]
       Date      Co #   Dr# Procedure   Diag       Units      Charges    Total Chgs

   1   06/02/08 11    3   99213      474.00        1.00        40.00       40.00
   2   06/02/08 11    3   87070      474.00        1.00        31.00       71.00




       Enter '?', '!', '?code' for Help, '?~' for Macros, or '%' for Standing Orders



Ready                                                          NUM      ↑↓◄►
```

Editing Prior Entries

In the unit exercises that follow, you will use the information provided to make changes to patient accounts.

EXERCISE 1: ADDING A DEPENDENT

WILLIAM SALVANI; ACCOUNT 312

GOAL(S): In this exercise, you will add a dependent to an existing account.

1. Before posting your entry, study the patient registration form in Figure 4-1. Answer the following questions.

   a. What is the relationship of the dependent to the guarantor? _____

   b. Does the dependent have extended information? _____

   c. Does the dependent have insurance? _____

Figure 4-1   Patient Registration Form – Kyle Salvani

Patient Registration Form

Sydney Carrington & Associates
34 Sycamore Street ● Madison, CA 95653

FOR OFFICE USE ONLY	
ACCOUNT NO.:	**312**
DOCTOR:	**#2**
BILL TYPE:	**11**
EXTENDED INFO.:	**0**

TODAY'S DATE: _06/02/2008_

PATIENT INFORMATION

Salvani	_Kyle_	_M._	
PATIENT LAST NAME	FIRST NAME	MI	SUFFIX

Floral City Elementary School
EMPLOYER OR SCHOOL NAME

MAILING ADDRESS	CITY	STATE ZIP CODE

Floral City | _CA_ | _94064_

EMPLOYER OR SCHOOL ADDRESS   CITY   STATE   ZIP CODE

_M_	_07/09/2002_	_Single_	_214-86-1392_
SEX (M/F)	DATE OF BIRTH	MARITAL STATUS	SOC. SEC. #

EMPLOYER OR SCHOOL PHONE NUMBER

Son	
HOME PHONE	RELATIONSHIP TO GUARANTOR

Thomas Bennett, MD
REFERRED BY

GUARANTOR INFORMATION

Salvani	_William_	_M_
RESPONSIBLE PARTY LAST NAME	FIRST NAME	MI SEX (M/F)

_02/26/1968_	_Married_	_158-23-4613_
DATE OF BIRTH	MARITAL STATUS	SOC. SEC. #

82 Cedar Brook Road – Apt 5A	
MAILING ADDRESS	STREET ADDRESS (IF DIFFERENT)

Better Business Bureau
EMPLOYER NAME

Sacramento	_CA_	_94056_
CITY	STATE	ZIP CODE

EMPLOYER ADDRESS

_(917) 826-1314_	_(917) 391-2873_
(AREA CODE) HOME PHONE	(AREA CODE) WORK PHONE

Sacramento	_CA_	_94056_
CITY	STATE	ZIP CODE

PRIMARY INSURANCE

Epsilon Life & Casualty
NAME OF PRIMARY INSURANCE COMPANY

Same
ADDRESS (IF DIFFERENT)

P.O. Box 189	
ADDRESS	

Same

Macon	_GA_	_31298_
CITY	STATE	ZIP CODE

_(800) 908-7654_	_158-23-4613_
CITY STATE ZIP CODE	

_17398QX_	_2003BR_
IDENTIFICATION #	GROUP NAME AND/OR #

PRIMARY INSURANCE PHONE NUMBER   SOC. SEC. #

Self

William Salvani	
INSURED PERSON'S NAME (IF DIFFERENT FROM THE RESPONSIBLE PARTY)	

WHAT IS THE RESPONSIBLE PARTY'S RELATIONSHIP TO THE INSURED?

SECONDARY INSURANCE

NAME OF SECONDARY INSURANCE COMPANY	ADDRESS (IF DIFFERENT)
ADDRESS	CITY STATE ZIP CODE
CITY STATE ZIP CODE	SECONDARY INSURANCE PHONE NUMBER SOC. SEC. #
IDENTIFICATION # GROUP NAME AND/OR #	WHAT IS THE RESPONSIBLE PARTY'S RELATIONSHIP TO THE INSURED?
INSURED PERSON'S NAME (IF DIFFERENT FROM THE RESPONSIBLE PARTY)	

I hereby consent for Sydney Carrington & Associates, P.A. to use or disclose my health information to carry out treatment, payment, and health care operations. I authorize the use of this signature on all insurance submissions. I understand that I am financially responsible for all charges whether or not paid by the insurance. I acknowledge receipt of the practice's privacy policy.

William Salvani (father)	_06/02/2008_
PATIENT SIGNATURE	DATE

2. Based on the information found on the patient registration form (Figure 4-1), add the dependent to Account 312. Compare your screen to Figure 4-2a. Process the dependent screen and add the extended information for Kyle Salvani. Compare your screen to Figure 4-2b.

Figure 4-2a Dependent Screen – Salvani

```
M Student: Lois Fitzpatrick                                                    _ □ X
File  Edit  View  Windows  Help

[toolbar icons]                                                  [toolbar icons]

   Account #: 312                    Dependent Information                   [Salvani]


          Dependent #                 : 2
          Dependent Last Name         : Salvani           Suffix : .....
          Dependent First Name        : Kyle              M.I. : M
          Dependent Date of Birth     : 07/09/2002
          Dependent Sex (M/F)         : M
          Relation to Guarantor       : C
          Social Security Number      : 214-86-1392
          Patient ID                  : ..............
          Patient ID 2                : ................
          Default Doctor #            :    2 Frances D Simpson M.D.
          Referring Doctor #          :   18 Thomas H Bennett M.D.
          Extended Information Level  : 2 Full
          WP File ID                  : C:wp312.2
          Marital Status              : S
          Race                        :
          Employment/Student Status   : F              Consent  : Y
          Date Became a Patient       : 06/02/2008     Deceased :
          E-Mail : ......................................................

            Enter (M)odify, (D)elete, (E)xtended, (L)ast Diags, (S)upp : .


Ready                                                        NUM     ↑↓⇦⇨
```

Figure 4-2b Extended Information – Kyle Salvani

```
M Student: Lois Fitzpatrick                                                    _ □ X
File  Edit  View  Windows  Help

[toolbar icons]                                                  [toolbar icons]


      Patient : Salvani,Kyle M                    Patient # : 312.2

                          * Extended Information *

   Employer / Co. : Floral City Elementary    Phone Number  : .........
   Address Line 1 : ......................    Identification : ..............
   Address Line 2 : ......................
   City           : Floral City
   State          : CA      Zip Code #    : 94064






                             * Comments *


   1:
   2:


                 Enter (M)odify or (D)elete : █


Ready                                                        NUM     ↑↓⇦⇨
```

EXERCISE 2: CHANGING A GUARANTOR'S LAST NAME, ADDING AN INSURANCE POLICY

ERIN KANTOR; ACCOUNT 313

Erin Kantor is an established patient. She has recently been married and called the office to update her account information.

GOAL(S): In this exercise, you will use the information provided to change a patient's last name and marital status and add insurance.

1. Erin's married name is Stein.
2. Modify her marital status. Compare your screen to Figure 4-3a.
3. Add **Pan American** as the insurance company. Her husband, Charles Stein, is the insured person. The insurance ID # is 5711434 and insured party ID # is 149187341. The group number is 648N. Charles and Erin reside at 30 Wilbur Street, Woodside, CA 98076. Charles's insurance coverage is through his employer, Statton Realty. Once the insurance information is entered, compare your screen to Figure 4-3b.
4. (**S**)et Coverage Priority after adding the insurance. Compare your screen to Figure 4-4.
5. Once the insurance information is processed, return to the account information screen and compare to Figure 4-5.

Figure 4-3a Account Information – Stein

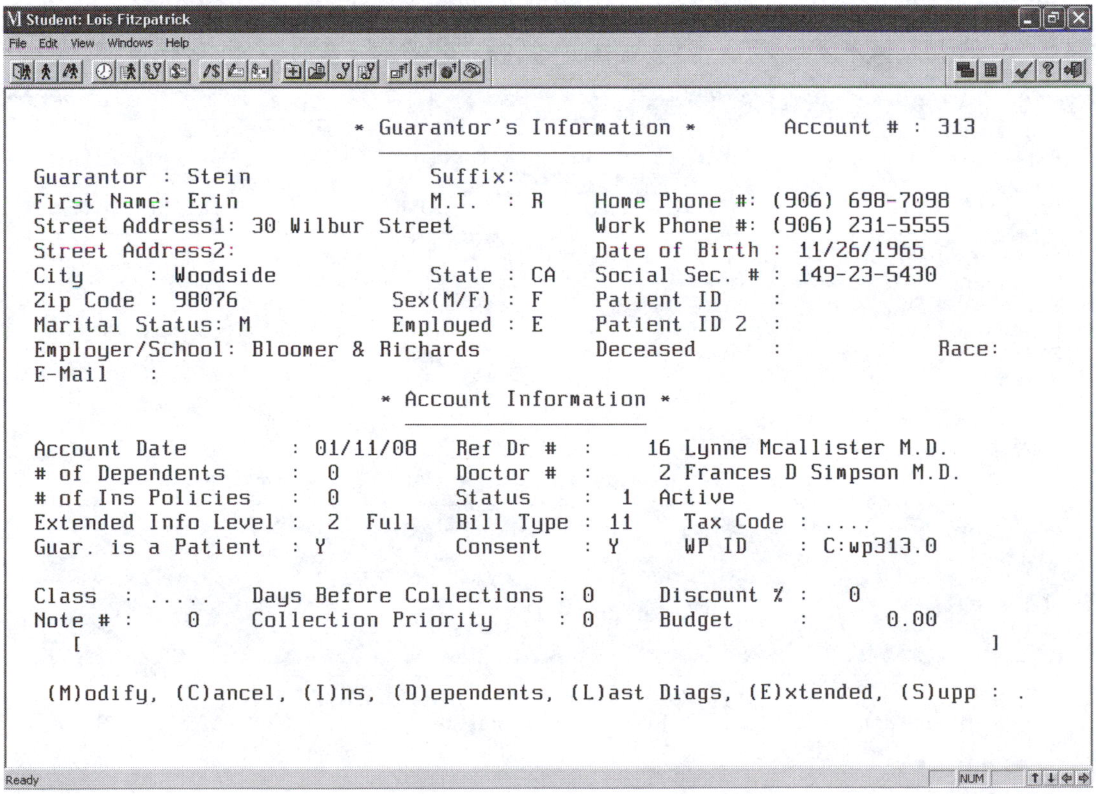
Student: Lois Fitzpatrick
File Edit View Windows Help

* Guarantor's Information * Account # : 313

Guarantor : Stein Suffix:
First Name: Erin M.I. : R Home Phone #: (906) 698-7098
Street Address1: 30 Wilbur Street Work Phone #: (906) 231-5555
Street Address2: Date of Birth : 11/26/1965
City : Woodside State : CA Social Sec. # : 149-23-5430
Zip Code : 98076 Sex(M/F) : F Patient ID :
Marital Status: M Employed : E Patient ID 2 :
Employer/School: Bloomer & Richards Deceased : Race:
E-Mail :

* Account Information *

Account Date : 01/11/08 Ref Dr # : 16 Lynne Mcallister M.D.
\# of Dependents : 0 Doctor # : 2 Frances D Simpson M.D.
\# of Ins Policies : 0 Status : 1 Active
Extended Info Level : 2 Full Bill Type : 11 Tax Code : ....
Guar. is a Patient : Y Consent : Y WP ID : C:wp313.0

Class : ..... Days Before Collections : 0 Discount % : 0
Note # : 0 Collection Priority : 0 Budget : 0.00
[ ]

(M)odify, (C)ancel, (I)ns, (D)ependents, (L)ast Diags, (E)xtended, (S)upp : .

Ready NUM

Figure 4-3b   Insurance Policy – Stein

```
M Student: Lois Fitzpatrick                                                          _ ☐ ✕
File  Edit  View  Windows  Help
☐✕ 🏃 🏃 ⏰ 🏃 💲 ⚡ ✏ ⊞ ⊞ 🗃 🗐 🗃 🗑 ●                                    🖥 ▦ ✓ ? ⇥

    Account #: 313                Insurance Policy Information                 [Stein]


    Policyholder   : 0       [Stein, Erin              ]
    Carrier Code   : PANAMC  [Pan American Health Ins. ]
    Plan #         : 7       Plan Code:              Form #   : 1    Fmt # : 1
    Plan Name      : Pan American Health Ins.        EMC ID 1 :
    Attention      :                                 EMC ID 2 :
    Street Address : 4567 Newberry Rd.               Deductible:      0.00
    City,State,Zip : Los Angeles     CA   98706      Program   : CI Commercial In
    Phone #        : (213) 456-7654   Class :        Assignment - Dr : Y  Pat : Y
    Group Number   : 648N                            Ins ID #  : 5711434

    Policy Dates - From :          To :              Copay Ext :     Ins Type: C1
         Insured Party #      : 18                   Rpt Group :
         Last Name or Company : Stein                         Suffix:
         First Name, M.I.     : Charles              Sex  : M  DOB :
         Address              : 30 Wilbur Street
         City,St,Zip          : Woodside        CA   98076
         Insured Party ID #   : 149187341             Phone :
         Insured's Employer   : Statton Realty
         Employer Ins Plan    : Y

                          Enter (M)odify or (D)elete : ▮


Ready                                                                   NUM   ↑↓⇦⇨
```

NOTE: Insured party numbers are assigned by the computer. The number assigned in this exercise may vary from that shown in Figure 4-4.

Figure 4-4   Coverage List – Stein

```
M Student: Lois Fitzpatrick                                                          _ ☐ ✕
File  Edit  View  Windows  Help
☐✕ 🏃 🏃 ⏰ 🏃 💲 ⚡ ✏ ⊞ ⊞ 🗃 🗐 🗃 🗑 ●                                    🖥 ▦ ✓ ? ⇥

    Patient #: 313.0          Insurance Coverage Priority             [Stein,Erin]
                                 [Guarantor List]
    Priority     Plan#      Plan Name              IPR          Relation to IPR

    Primary  :   7.0        Pan American Health Ins.  Stein,Charles          W
    Secondary:   ........                                                    .
    Third    :   ........                                                    .
    Fourth   :   ........                                                    .
    Fifth    :   ........                                                    .
    Sixth    :   ........                                                    .
    Seventh  :   ........                                                    .

    [Policies]
    Plan#     Plan Name           Holder     User Note      Insured Party

        7.0   Pan American Health  Erin                      Stein,Charles




        (M)aintain List, (C)lear List, (U)se Guarantor List, or <PROCESS> : .


Ready                                                                   NUM   ↑↓⇦⇨
```

Figure 4-5 Account Information – Stein

```
M Student: Lois Fitzpatrick                                                    _ ⊡ ✕
File  Edit  View  Windows  Help
⬚⬚ ⬚⬚⬚ ⬚⬚⬚⬚ ⬚⬚⬚⬚ ⬚⬚⬚⬚ ⬚⬚⬚⬚⬚                                     ⬚⬚  ✓⬚⬚

                         * Guarantor's Information *         Account # : 313

  Guarantor : Stein              Suffix:
  First Name: Erin               M.I.  : R   Home Phone #: (906) 698-7098
  Street Address1: 30 Wilbur Street          Work Phone #: (906) 231-5555
  Street Address2:                           Date of Birth : 11/26/1965
  City    : Woodside          State : CA   Social Sec. # : 149-23-5430
  Zip Code : 98076           Sex(M/F) : F   Patient ID    :
  Marital Status: M          Employed : E   Patient ID 2  :
  Employer/School: Bloomer & Richards        Deceased      :          Race:
  E-Mail   :
                          * Account Information *

  Account Date       : 01/11/08   Ref Dr # :   16 Lynne Mcallister M.D.
  # of Dependents    :  0         Doctor # :    2 Frances D Simpson M.D.
  # of Ins Policies  :  1         Status   :  1 Active
  Extended Info Level :  2  Full  Bill Type : 11   Tax Code : ....
  Guar. is a Patient :  Y         Consent  :  Y   WP ID    : C:wp313.0


  Class  : .....   Days Before Collections : 0   Discount % :   0
  Note # :    0    Collection Priority     : 0   Budget     :     0.00
     [                                                              ]

   (M)odify, (C)ancel, (I)ns, (D)ependents, (L)ast Diags, (E)xtended, (S)upp : .


Ready                                                           NUM    ↑↓⇦⇨
```

EXERCISE 3: CHANGING A GUARANTOR'S ADDRESS, EMPLOYER, AND EXTENDED INFORMATION

CARMEN FUENTAS; ACCOUNT 314

Carmen Fuentas calls to say she has moved and changed her employment.

GOAL(S): Using the information Carmen provides, you will update her address, employment information, and telephone numbers.

1. Carmen has moved to 83 Hyatt Court, Madison, CA 95653.

2. Carmen now works at Regency Enterprises, 632 Walton Avenue, Madison, CA 95653.

3. Carmen's home phone number is (916) 810-4385. Her work phone number is (916) 539-2810. Compare your screen to Figures 4-6 and 4-7.

Figure 4-6   Account Information – Fuentas

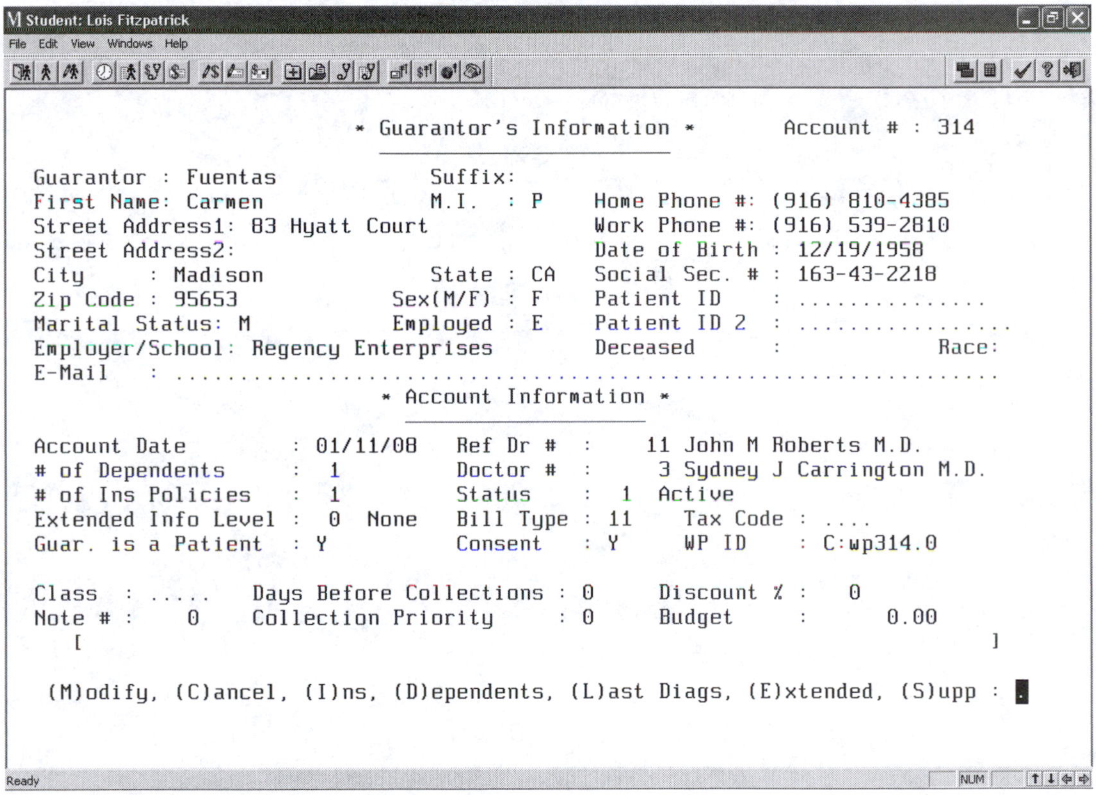

Figure 4-7   Extended Information – Fuentas

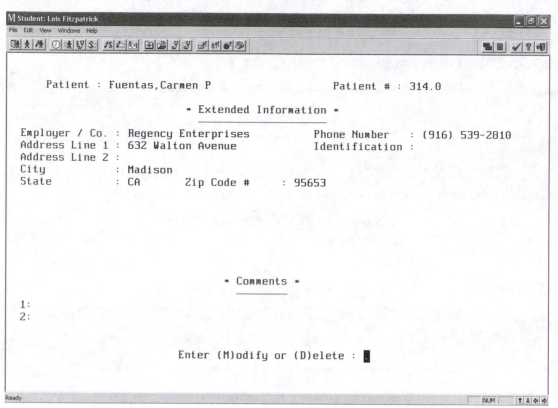

EXERCISE 4: CORRECTING A POSTED PROCEDURE AND DIAGNOSIS

MARGARET MORGAN; ACCOUNT 315

When Margaret was seen by the doctor on 06/02/2008, the procedure code 99213 was mistakenly entered instead of the code 99214 and the diagnosis, chest pain, was not used for the x-ray.

GOAL(S): Using the information provided above and the encounter form (Figure 4-8), you will edit the activity to correct the procedure code and add the chest pain diagnosis code to the visit. Enter the chest pain diagnosis with the X-ray Chest PA & Lat procedure. Compare your screen to Figures 4-9 and 4-10.

Figure 4-8 Encounter Form – Morgan

Sydney Carrington & Associates P.A.
34 Sycamore Street Suite 300
Madison, CA 95653

Date: 06/02/2008   Voucher No.: 3280

Time: 09:00

Patient: Margaret Morgan   Patient No: 315.0
Guarantor: Margaret Morgan   Doctor: 3 – S. Carrington

CPT	DESCRIPTION	FEE
OFFICE/HOSPITAL CONSULTS		
☐ 99201	Office New:Focused Hx-Exam	
☐ 99202	Office New:Expanded Hx.Exam	
☐ 99211	Office Estb:Min./None Hx-Exa	
☐ 99212	Office Estb:Focused Hx-Exam	
☐ 99213	Office Estb:Expanded Hx-Exa	
☒ 99214	Office Estb:Detailed Hx-Exa	$50.00
☐ 99215	Office Estb:Comprhn Hx-Exam	
☐ 99221	Hosp. Initial:Comprh Hx-	
☐ 99223	Hosp. Ini:Comprh Hx-Exam/Hi	
☐ 99231	Hosp. Subsequent: S-Fwd	
☐ 99232	Hosp. Subsequent: Comprhn Hx	
☐ 99233	Hosp. Subsequent: Ex/Hi	
☐ 99238	Hospital Visit Discharge Ex	
☐ 99371	Telephone Consult - Simple	
☐ 99372	Telephone Consult - Intermed	
☐ 99373	Telephone Consult - Complex	
☐ 90840	Counseling - 25 minutes	
☐ 90806	Counseling - 50 minutes	
☐ 90865	Counseling - Special Interview	
IMMUNIZATIONS/INJECTIONS		
☐ 90585	BCG Vaccine	
☐ 90659	Influenza Virus Vaccine	
☐ 90701	Immunization-DTP	
☐ 90702	DT Vaccine	
☐ 90703	Tetanus Toxoids	
☐ 90732	Pneumococcal Vaccine	
☐ 90746	Hepatitis B Vaccine	
☐ 90749	Immunization: Unlisted	

CPT	DESCRIPTION	FEE
LABORATORY/RADIOLOGY		
☐ 81000	Urinalysis	
☐ 81002	Urinalysis; Pregnancy Test	
☐ 82951	Glucose Tolerance Test	
☐ 84478	Triglycerides	
☐ 84550	Uric Acid: Blood Chemistry	
☐ 84830	Ovulation Test	
☐ 85014	Hematocrit	
☐ 85032	Hemogram, Complete Blood Wk	
☐ 86403	Particle Agglutination Test	
☐ 86485	Skin Test; Candida	
☐ 86580	TB Intradermal Test	
☐ 86585	TB Tine Test	
☐ 87070	Culture	
☐ 70190	X-Ray; Optic Foramina	
☐ 70210	X-Ray Sinuses Complete	
☐ 71010	Radiological Exam Ent Spine	
☒ 71020	X-Ray Chest Pa & Lat	$58.00
☐ 72050	X-Ray Spine, Cerv (4 views)	
☐ 72090	X-Ray Spine; Scoliosis Ex	
☐ 72110	Spine, lumbosacral; a/p & Lat	
☐ 73030	Shoulder-Comp, min w/ 2vws	
☐ 73070	Elbow, anteropost & later vws	
☐ 73120	X-Ray; Hand, 2 views	
☐ 73560	X-Ray, Knee, 1 or 2 views	
☐ 74022	X-Ray; Abdomen, Complete	
☐ 75552	Cardiac Magnetic Res Img	
☐ 76020	X-Ray; Bone Age Studies	
☐ 77054	Mammary Ductogram Complete	
☐ 78465	Myocardial Perfusion Img	

CPT	DESCRIPTION	FEE
PROCEDURES/TESTS		
☐ 00452	Anesthesia for Rad Surgery	
☐ 11100	Skin Biopsy	
☐ 15852	Dressing Change	
☐ 29075	Cast Appl. - Lower Arm	
☐ 29530	Strapping of Knee	
☐ 29705	Removal/Revis of Cast w/Exa	
☐ 53670	Catheterization Incl. Suppl	
☐ 57452	Colposcopy	
☐ 57505	ECC	
☐ 69420	Myringotomy	
☐ 92081	Visual Field Examination	
☐ 92100	Serial Tonometry Exam	
☐ 92120	Tonography	
☐ 92552	Pure Tone Audiometry	
☐ 92567	Tympanometry	
☐ 93000	Electrocardiogram	
☐ 93015	Exercise Stress Test (ETT)	
☐ 93017	ETT Tracing Only	
☐ 93040	Electrocardiogram - Rhythm	
☐ 96100	Psychological Testing	
☐ 99000	Specimen Handling	
☐ 99058	Office Emergency Care	
☐ 99070	Surgical Tray - Misc.	
☐ 99080	Special Reports of Med Rec	
☐ 99195	Phlebotomy	
☐ _____	_____	
☐ _____	_____	
☐ _____	_____	

ICD-9 CODE DIAGNOSIS		
☐ 009.0	Infect. colitis, enteritis, & gastroenteritis	
☐ 133.0	Scabies	
☐ 174.9	Breast Cancer, Female, Unspecified	
☐ 185	Malignant neoplasm of prostate	
☐ 250.00	Diabetes Mellitus w/o mention of Complication	
☐ 272.4	Hyperlipidemia	
☐ 282.5	Anemia, Sickle-cell Trait	
☐ 282.60	Sickle-cell disease, unspecified	
☒ 285.9	Anemia, Unspecified	
☐ 300.4	Dysthymic disorder	
☐ 340	Multiple Sclerosis	
☐ 342.90	Hemiplegia - Unspec.	
☐ 346.90	Migraine, unspecified	
☐ 352.9	Unspecified disorder of cranial nerves	
☐ 354.0	Carpal Tunnel Syndrome	
☐ 355.0	Sciatic Nerve Root Lesion	
☐ 366.9	Cataract	
☐ 386.00	Menier's disease, unspecified	
☐ 401.1	Essential Hypertension, Benign	
☐ 414.9	Ischemic Heart Disease	
☐ 428.0	Congestive Heart Failure (CHF), unspecified	

ICD-9 CODE DIAGNOSIS		
☐ 435.0	Basilar Artery Syndrome	
☐ 440.0	Atherosclerosis	
☐ 442.81	Carotid Artery	
☐ 460	Common Cold (Acute Nasopharyngitis)	
☐ 461.9	Acute Sinusitis	
☐ 474.00	Chronic Tonsillitis & Adenoiditis	
☐ 477.9	Allergic Rhinitis, Cause Unspecified	
☐ 487.0	Influenza with pneumonia	
☐ 496	Chronic Airway Obstruction	
☐ 522.0	Pulpitis	
☐ 524.60	Temporo-Mandibular Joint Disorder - Unspec.	
☐ 536.8	Stomach Pain	
☐ 553.3	Hiatal Hernia	
☐ 564.1	Spastic Colon	
☐ 574.40	Chronic Hepatitis, Unspecified	
☐ 571.5	Cirrhosis of Liver w/o mention of alcohol	
☐ 573.3	Hepatitis	
☐ 575.2	Obstruction of Gallbladder	
☐ 648.20	Anemia - Compl. Pregnancy	
☐ 715.90	Osteoarthritis - Unspec.	
☐ 721.3	Lumbar Osteo/Spondylarthrit	

ICD-9 CODE DIAGNOSIS		
☐ 724.2	Pain: Lower Back	
☐ 727.67	Rupture of Achilles Tendon	
☐ 780.1	Hallucinations	
☐ 780.3	Convulsions, Other	
☐ 780.50	Sleep Disturbances, Unspecified	
☐ 783.0	Anorexia	
☐ 783.1	Abnormal Weight Gain	
☐ 783.21	Abnormal Weight Loss	
☐ 823.80	Fractured Tibia	
☐ 823.81	Fractured Fibula	
☐ 831.00	Dislocated Shoulder, Closed, Unspecified	
☐ 835.00	Dislocated Hip, Closed, Unspecified	
☐ 842.00	Sprained Wrist, Unspecified Site	(786.50)
☐ 845.00	Sprained Ankle, Unspecified Site	
☐ 919.5	Insect Bite, Nonvenomous	
☐ 921.1	Contus Eyelid/Perioc Area	
☐ v16.3	Fam. Hist of Breast Cancer	
☐ v17.4	Fam. Hist of Cardiovasc Dis	
☐ v20.2	Well Child	
☐ v22.0	Pregnancy - First Normal	
☐ v22.1	Pregnancy - Normal	

Previous Balance	Today's Charges	Total Due	Amount Paid	New Balance
0	108.00	108.00	0	108.00

Follow Up

PRN _____ Weeks _____ Months _____ Units _____

Next Appointment Date: _____ Time: _____

I hereby authorize release of any information acquired in the course of examination or treatment and allow a photocopy of my signature to be used.

_____

Figure 4-9 Corrected Procedure Code

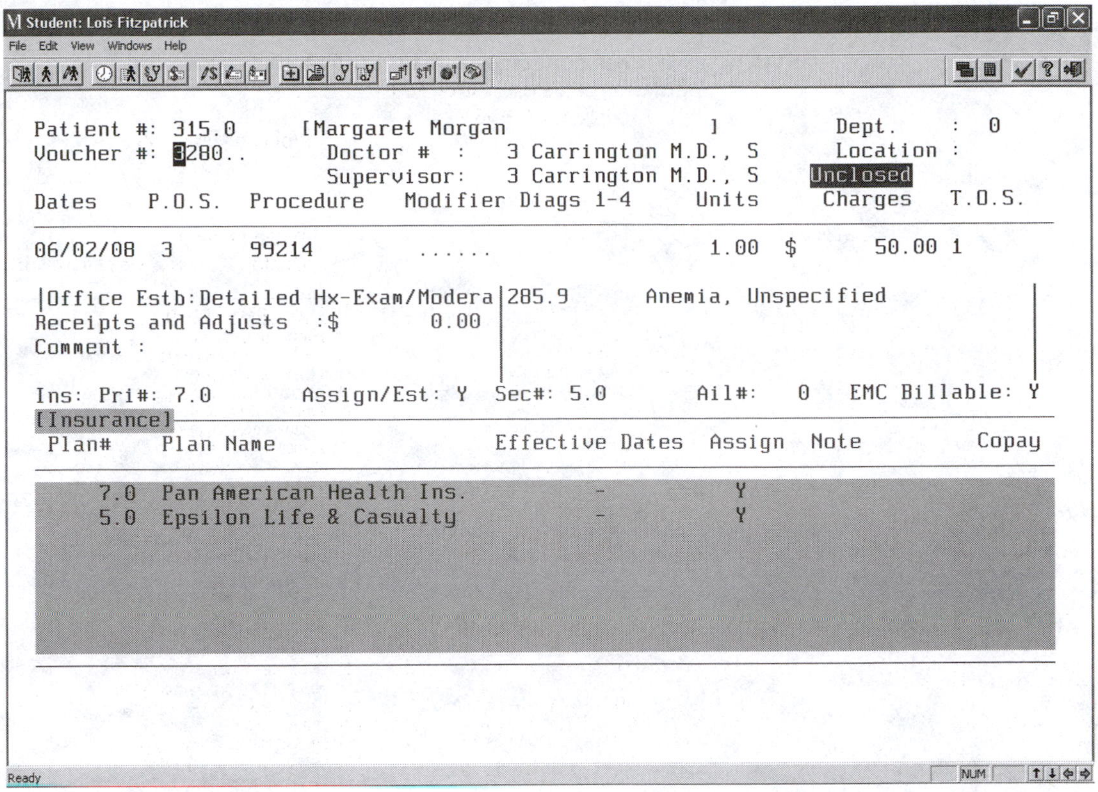

Figure 4-10 Corrected Diagnosis Code

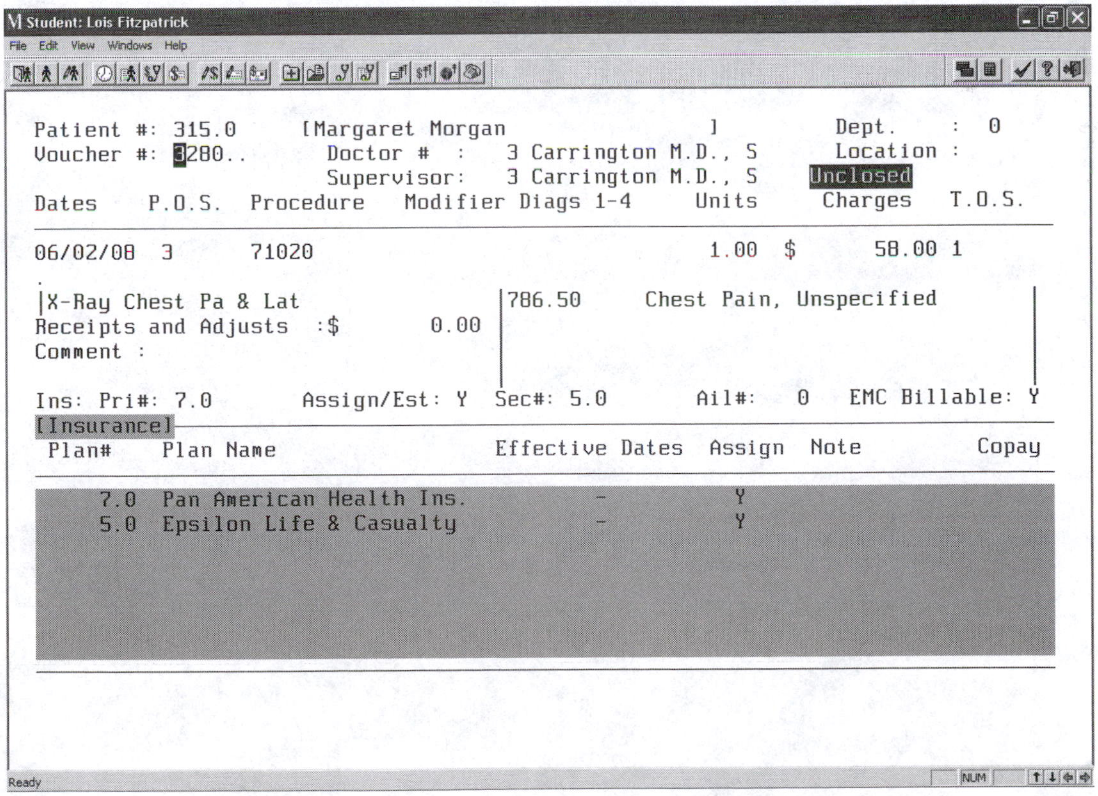

EXERCISE 5: ADDING A DIAGNOSIS TO A POSTED PROCEDURE

SHARON BARKER; ACCOUNT 316

An additional diagnosis code is to be added to Sharon Barker's account for the 06/02/2008 visit.

GOAL(S): Using the information provided, you will edit activity to add a second diagnosis code, 724.2 (Pain: Lower Back) to Sharon Barker's account for all three procedures performed. Compare your screen to Figures 4-11, 4-12, and 4-13.

Figure 4-11 Additional Diagnosis Code – 724.2

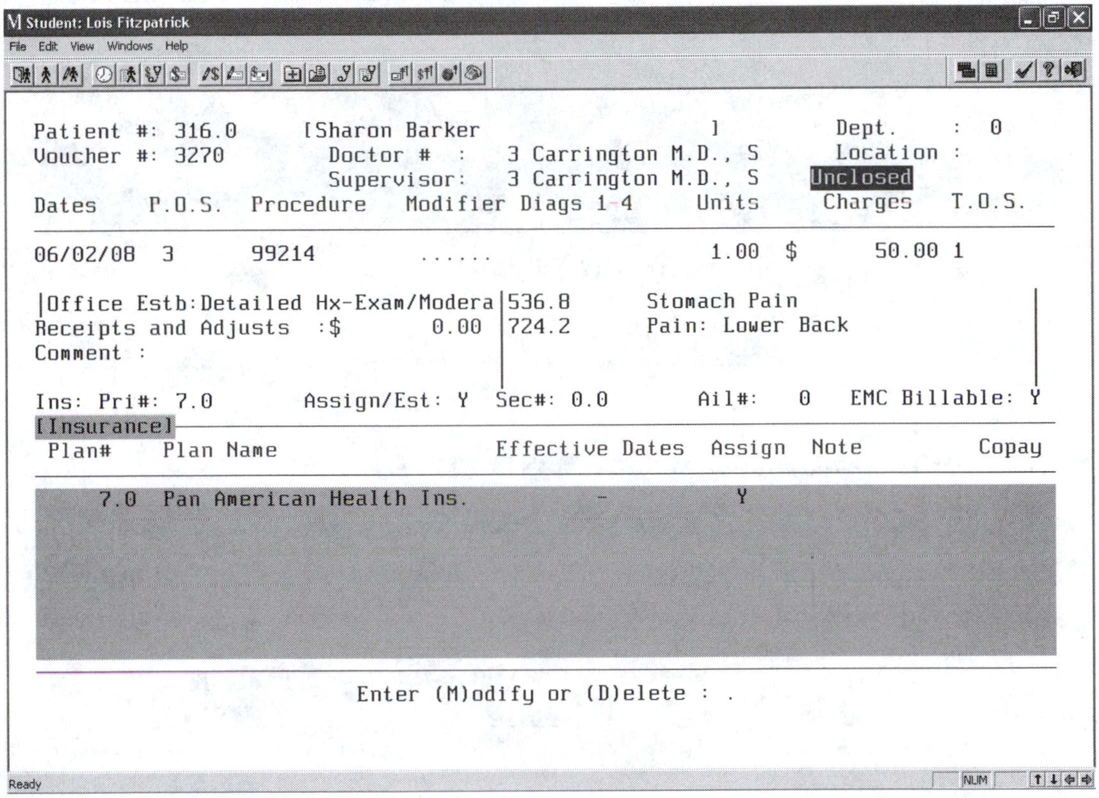

Figure 4-12   Second Procedure with Added Diagnosis Code

```
M Student: Lois Fitzpatrick                                              _ □ ☒
File  Edit  View  Windows  Help

 ▨▸▨ ⦾▸▨⦿▨  ▨◿▨  ▨▨ ▨▨ ▨▨▨◉▨

   Patient #: 316.0     [Sharon Barker              ]      Dept.    :  0
   Voucher #: 3270         Doctor #  :   3 Carrington M.D., S    Location :
                           Supervisor:   3 Carrington M.D., S   Unclosed
   Dates     P.O.S.   Procedure   Modifier Diags 1-4    Units    Charges   T.O.S.
  ─────────────────────────────────────────────────────────────────────────
   06/02/08  3         81000        ......            1.00  $      8.00 1

   |Urinalysis by dip stick or tablet  |536.8    Stomach Pain
   Receipts and Adjusts   :$      0.00 |724.2    Pain: Lower Back
   Comment :

   Ins: Pri#: 7.0       Assign/Est: Y  Sec#: 0.0      Ail#:   0   EMC Billable: Y
   [Insurance]
     Plan#    Plan Name              Effective Dates  Assign  Note       Copay
  ┌──────────────────────────────────────────────────────────────────────────┐
  │    7.0  Pan American Health Ins.          -        Y                      │
  │                                                                            │
  │                                                                            │
  │                                                                            │
  │                                                                            │
  └──────────────────────────────────────────────────────────────────────────┘

                   Enter (M)odify or (D)elete : .

Ready                                                        NUM      ↑↓⇐⇒
```

Figure 4-13   Final procedure with diagnosis 724.2 added

```
M Student: Lois Fitzpatrick                                              _ □ ☒
File  Edit  View  Windows  Help

 ▨▸▨ ⦾▸▨⦿▨  ▨◿▨  ▨▨ ▨▨ ▨▨▨◉▨

   Patient #: 316.0     [Sharon Barker              ]      Dept.    :  0
   Voucher #: 3270         Doctor #  :   3 Carrington M.D., S    Location :
                           Supervisor:   3 Carrington M.D., S   Unclosed
   Dates     P.O.S.   Procedure   Modifier Diags 1-4    Units    Charges   T.O.S.
  ─────────────────────────────────────────────────────────────────────────
   06/02/08  3         87070        ......            1.00  $     31.00 1

   |Culture                            |536.8    Stomach Pain
   Receipts and Adjusts   :$      0.00 |724.2    Pain: Lower Back
   Comment :

   Ins: Pri#: 7.0       Assign/Est: Y  Sec#: 0.0      Ail#:   0   EMC Billable: Y
   [Insurance]
     Plan#    Plan Name              Effective Dates  Assign  Note       Copay
  ┌──────────────────────────────────────────────────────────────────────────┐
  │    7.0  Pan American Health Ins.          -        Y                      │
  │                                                                            │
  │                                                                            │
  │                                                                            │
  │                                                                            │
  └──────────────────────────────────────────────────────────────────────────┘

                   Enter (M)odify or (D)elete : .

Ready                                                        NUM      ↑↓⇐⇒
```

U N I T 5

Office Management/
Appointment Scheduling

In the unit exercises that follow, you will use the information provided to schedule individual and multiple appointments, post procedures and schedule follow-up appointments, cancel and reschedule appointments, and print daily list of appointments and hospital rounds report.

EXERCISE 1: SCHEDULING APPOINTMENTS

CATHERINE VIAJO

GOAL(S): Schedule an individual appointment in two weeks.

Catherine Viajo calls for an appointment for a general check-up in two weeks. She needs an early morning appointment.

1. Using the information above, schedule Catherine's appointment with Dr. Simpson at 9:30. Compare your screen to Figure 5-1.

Figure 5-1   Appointment – Viajo

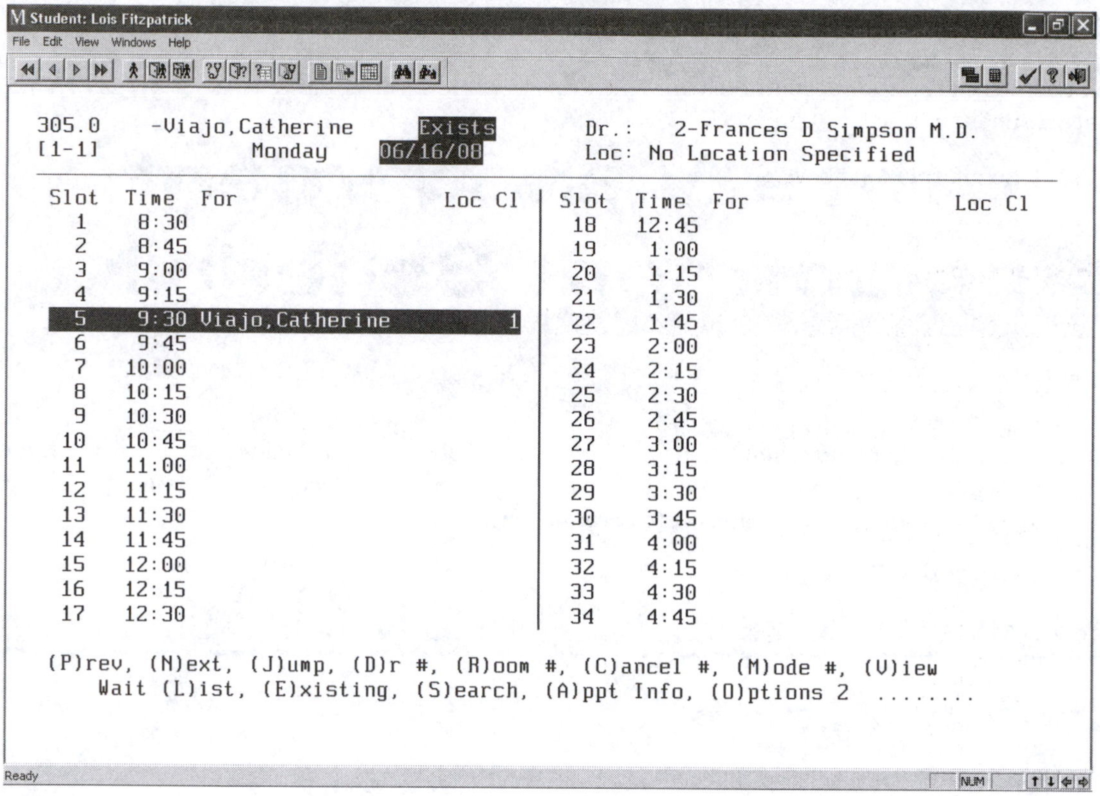

```
M Student: Lois Fitzpatrick                                                    _ □ X
File  Edit  View  Windows  Help

  ◀◀ ◀ ▶ ▶▶   👤 📷 📖   📋 📑 📝 📘   📄 📇 🖥   🔍 🔎                        🗐 🖥 ✔ ? 🔚

    305.0      -Viajo,Catherine      Exists        Dr.:    2-Frances D Simpson M.D.
    [1-1]                 Monday     06/16/08       Loc: No Location Specified
    ─────────────────────────────────────────────────────────────────────────────
    Slot  Time  For                Loc Cl    Slot  Time  For                Loc Cl
      1   8:30                                 18  12:45
      2   8:45                                 19   1:00
      3   9:00                                 20   1:15
      4   9:15                                 21   1:30
      5   9:30 Viajo,Catherine          1     22   1:45
      6   9:45                                 23   2:00
      7  10:00                                 24   2:15
      8  10:15                                 25   2:30
      9  10:30                                 26   2:45
     10  10:45                                 27   3:00
     11  11:00                                 28   3:15
     12  11:15                                 29   3:30
     13  11:30                                 30   3:45
     14  11:45                                 31   4:00
     15  12:00                                 32   4:15
     16  12:15                                 33   4:30
     17  12:30                                 34   4:45

    (P)rev, (N)ext, (J)ump, (D)r #, (R)oom #, (C)ancel #, (M)ode #, (V)iew
        Wait (L)ist, (E)xisting, (S)earch, (A)ppt Info, (O)ptions 2  ........

Ready                                                            NUM      ↑↓◀▶
```

DAVID FUENTAS

GOAL(S): Schedule an individual appointment with multiple slots for Wednesday, June 18.

David Fuentas calls for an appointment for a personal consult on June 18 at 11:30 with Dr. Carrington. The appointment will be for 30 minutes.

1. Using the information above, schedule David's appointment. Compare your screen to Figure 5-2.

Figure 5-2 Appointment – Fuentas

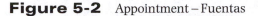

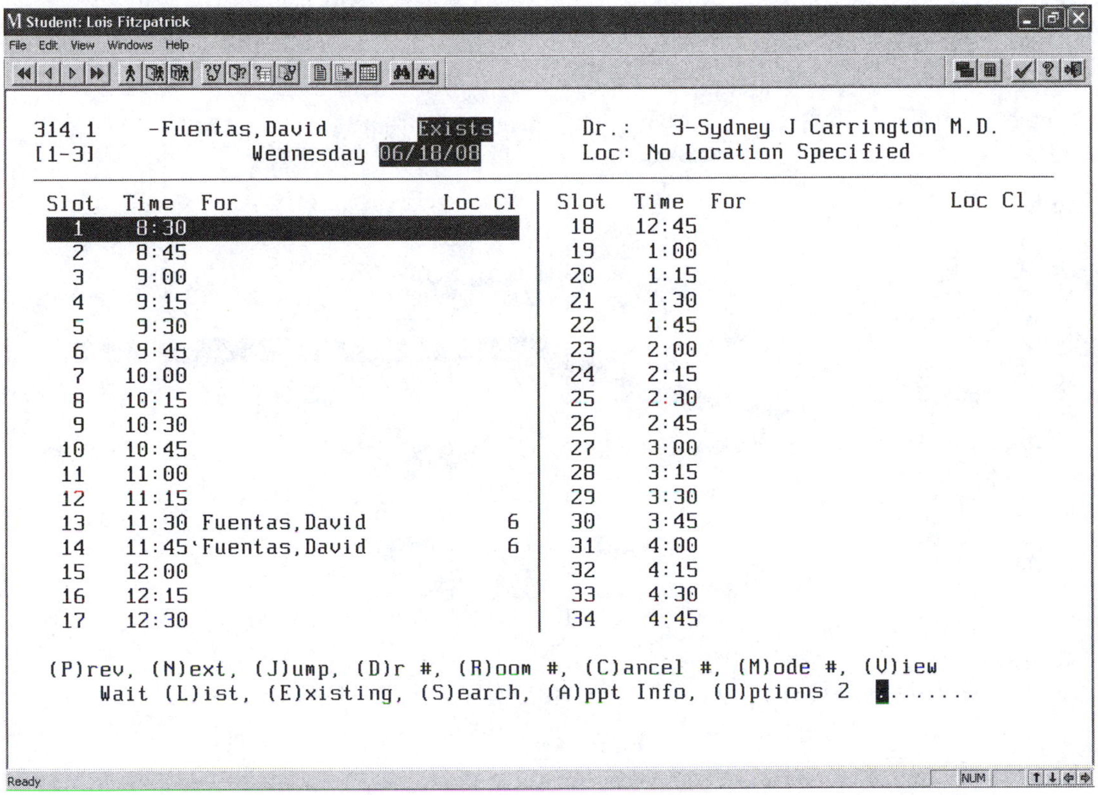

```
M Student: Lois Fitzpatrick                                               _ ☐ ✕
File  Edit  View  Windows  Help

  314.1     -Fuentas,David      Exists      Dr.:   3-Sydney J Carrington M.D.
  [1-3]               Wednesday 06/18/08     Loc: No Location Specified

  Slot  Time  For            Loc Cl    Slot  Time  For            Loc Cl
   1     8:30                            18    12:45
   2     8:45                            19     1:00
   3     9:00                            20     1:15
   4     9:15                            21     1:30
   5     9:30                            22     1:45
   6     9:45                            23     2:00
   7    10:00                            24     2:15
   8    10:15                            25     2:30
   9    10:30                            26     2:45
  10    10:45                            27     3:00
  11    11:00                            28     3:15
  12    11:15                            29     3:30
  13    11:30 Fuentas,David        6     30     3:45
  14    11:45'Fuentas,David       6     31     4:00
  15    12:00                            32     4:15
  16    12:15                            33     4:30
  17    12:30                            34     4:45

  (P)rev, (N)ext, (J)ump, (D)r #, (R)oom #, (C)ancel #, (M)ode #, (V)iew
       Wait (L)ist, (E)xisting, (S)earch, (A)ppt Info, (O)ptions 2 ■.......

Ready                                                              NUM    ↑↓⇠⇢
```

MARGARET MORGAN

GOAL(S): Schedule a recheck appointment.

Margaret Morgan needs to schedule a recheck appointment for June 17 with Dr. Carrington.

1. Using the information above, schedule Margaret's appointment at 2:00. Compare your screen to Figure 5-3.

Figure 5-3 Appointment – Morgan

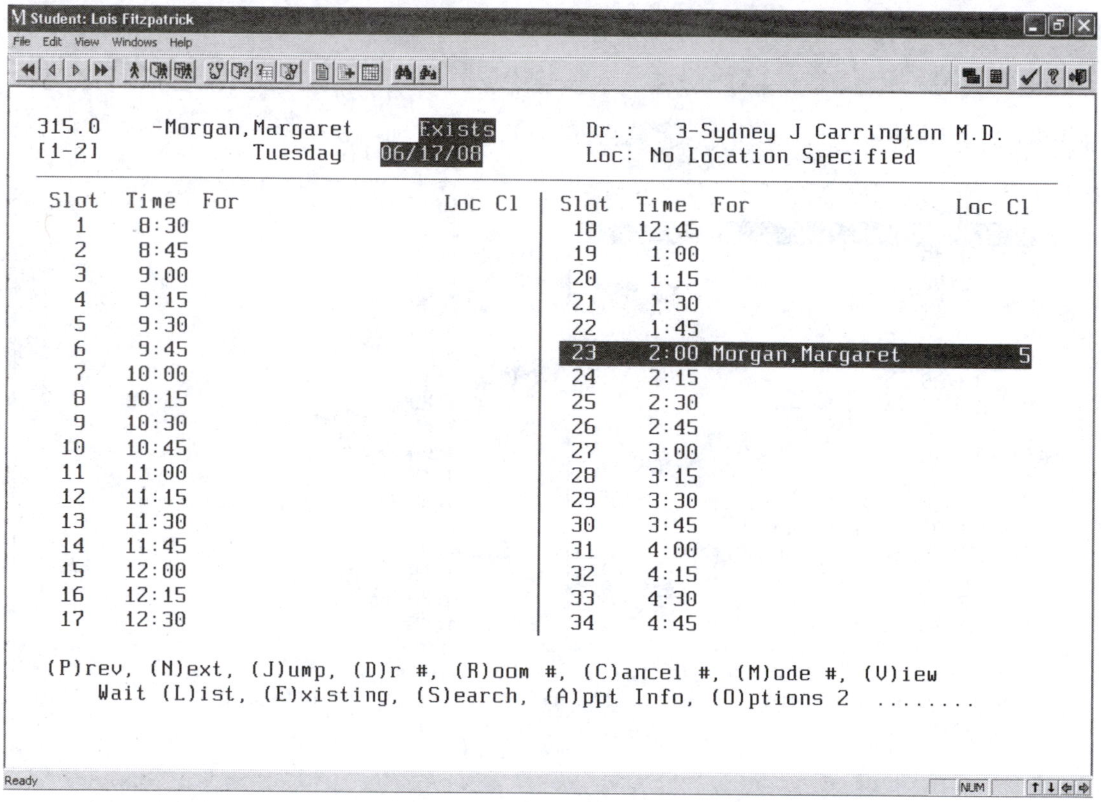

EXERCISE 2: SCHEDULE AN APPOINTMENT (NEXT DAY)

CHRISTINE CUSACK

GOAL(S): Schedule an individual appointment for the next day.

Christine Cusack calls for an appointment for a prenatal exam for tomorrow. She would like an early afternoon appointment.

1. Using the information above, schedule Christine's appointment with Dr. Monroe at 1:00. Compare your screen to Figure 5-4.

Figure 5-4   Appointment – Cusack

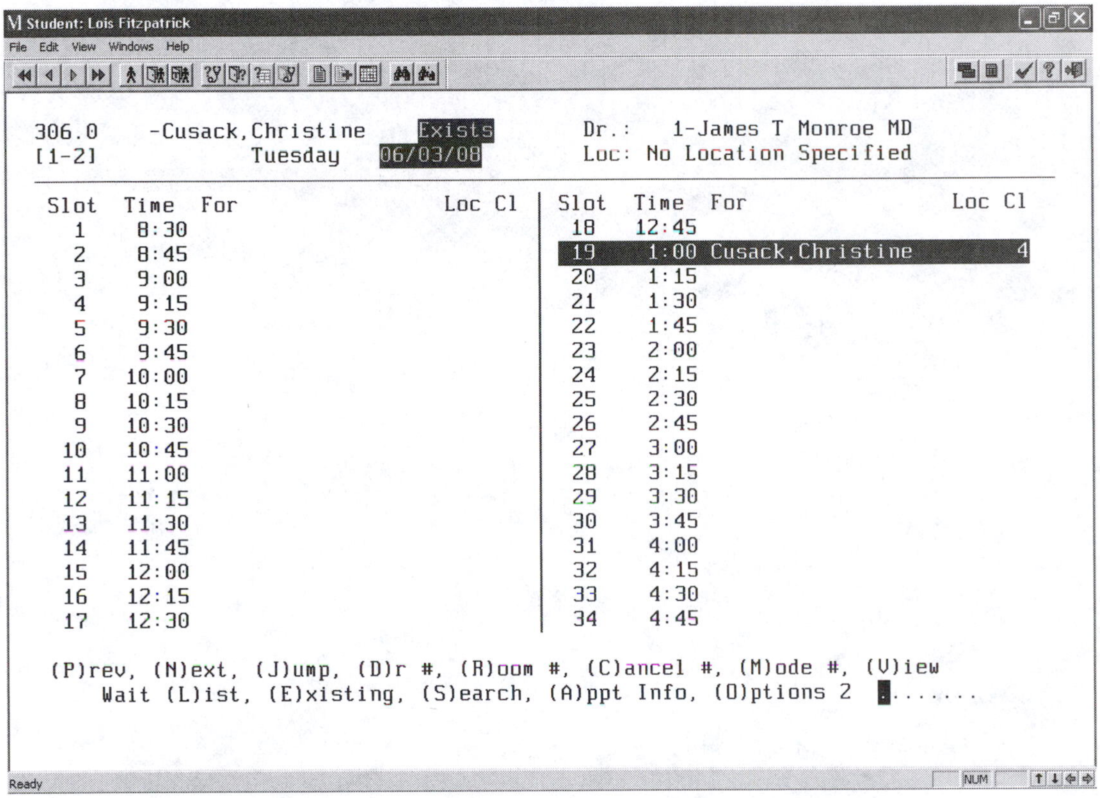

EXERCISE 3: SCHEDULE A MULTI-SLOT APPOINTMENT

JOHN WYATT

GOAL(S): Schedule an appointment with multiple slots in three weeks.

John Wyatt calls for an appointment for a personal consult in three weeks. He needs a late afternoon appointment.

1. Using the information above, schedule John's appointment with Dr. Monroe at 4:00 for 30 minutes. Compare your screen to Figure 5-5.

Figure 5-5   Appointment – Wyatt

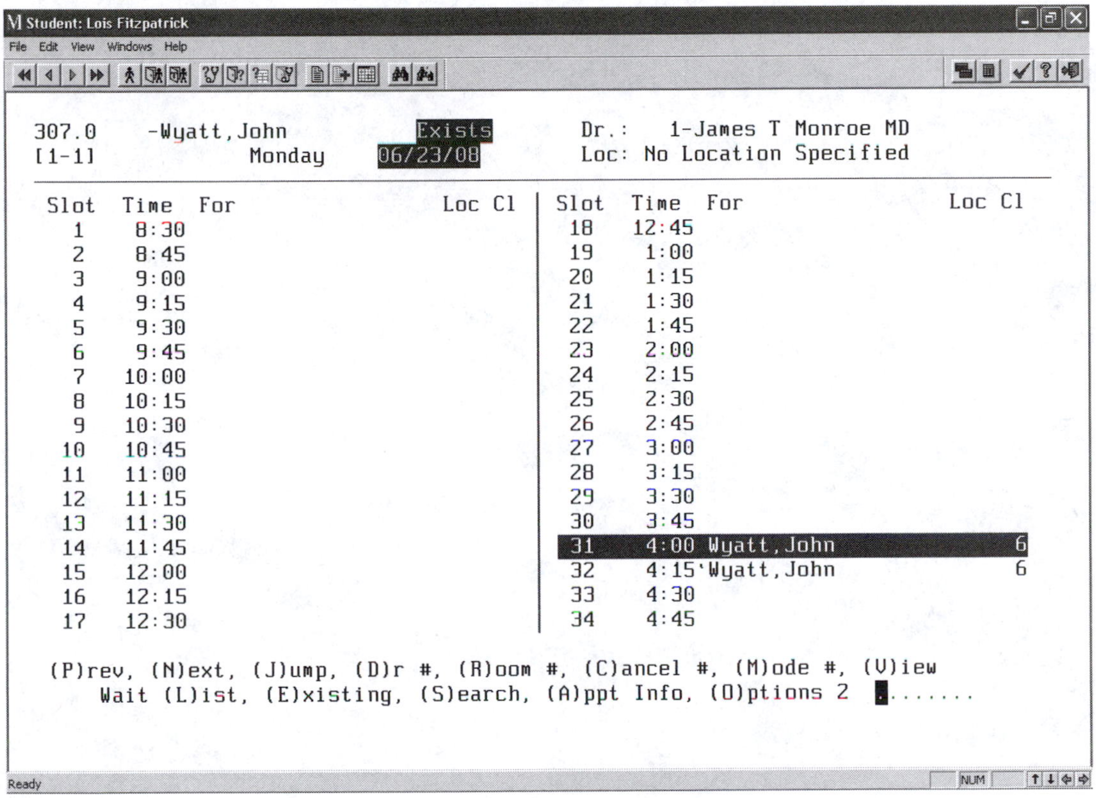

EXERCISE 4: SCHEDULE ANOTHER MULTI-SLOT APPOINTMENT

LINDA FROST

GOAL(S): Schedule an appointment with multiple slots for Wednesday, 06/04/2008.

Linda Frost needs to have an x-ray done on her wrist. She cannot come into the office until Wednesday. She would like a morning appointment.

1. Using the information above, schedule Linda's appointment with Dr. Carrington at 10:00 for 30 minutes. Compare your screen to Figure 5-6.

Figure 5-6 Appointment – Frost

```
M Student: Lois Fitzpatrick                                          _ 🗗 ✕
File  Edit  View  Windows  Help
◀◀ ◀ ▶ ▶▶   🕴📑📑  🔁📑📑📑  📄📑📰  📷📷                    📑📑 ✓ ? 📑

   308.1      -Frost,Linda        Exists      Dr.:   3-Sydney J Carrington M.D.
   [1-3]               Wednesday 06/04/08      Loc: No Location Specified

   Slot  Time  For              Loc Cl  │  Slot  Time  For              Loc Cl
     1   8:30                            │   18   12:45
     2   8:45                            │   19   1:00
     3   9:00                            │   20   1:15
     4   9:15                            │   21   1:30
     5   9:30                            │   22   1:45
     6   9:45                            │   23   2:00
     7   10:00 Frost,Linda         7     │   24   2:15
     8   10:15'Frost,Linda        7      │   25   2:30
     9   10:30                            │   26   2:45
    10   10:45                            │   27   3:00
    11   11:00                            │   28   3:15
    12   11:15                            │   29   3:30
    13   11:30                            │   30   3:45
    14   11:45                            │   31   4:00
    15   12:00                            │   32   4:15
    16   12:15                            │   33   4:30
    17   12:30                            │   34   4:45

   (P)rev, (N)ext, (J)ump, (D)r #, (R)oom #, (C)ancel #, (M)ode #, (V)iew
        Wait (L)ist, (E)xisting, (S)earch, (A)ppt Info, (O)ptions 2  ........

Ready                                                         NUM    ↑↓◀▶
```

EXERCISE 5: SCHEDULE AN APPOINTMENT CONFLICT

JUAN PEREZ

GOAL(S): Schedule an appointment for Wednesday, 06/04/2008, creating an appointment conflict.

Juan Perez calls to schedule a general check-up at 10:15 on Wednesday, 06/04/2008. He would like to see Dr. Carrington.

1. Using the information above, schedule Juan's appointment, accepting the conflict. Compare your screen to Figure 5-7.

Figure 5-7 Appointment Conflict

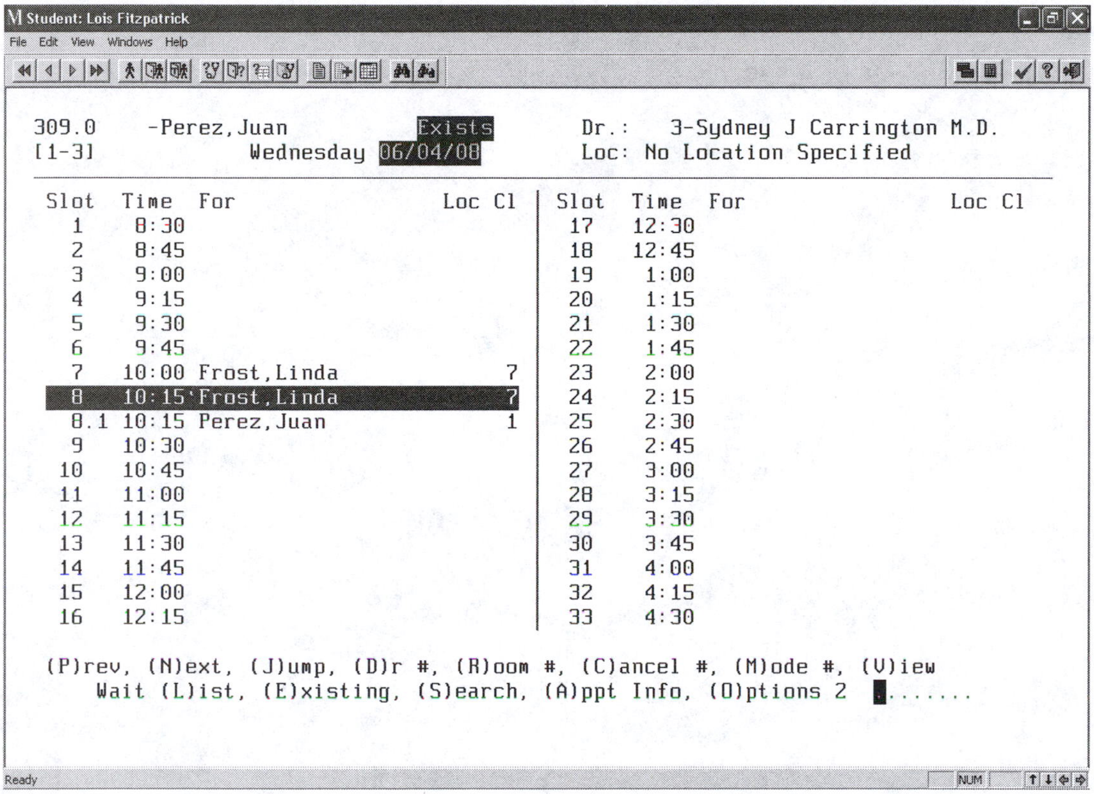

EXERCISE 6: SCHEDULE A DIFFERENT DOCTOR

MATTHEW NOONAN

GOAL(S): Schedule an appointment with a different doctor.

Matthew Noonan needs an appointment for an annual check-up in two weeks and he would like to see Dr. Monroe.

1. Key "?NOONAN" to retrieve Matthew Noonan by name.

2. Using the information above, schedule Matthew's appointment with Dr. Monroe at 3:30. Compare your screen to Figure 5-8.

Figure 5-8   Appointment with Dr. Monroe

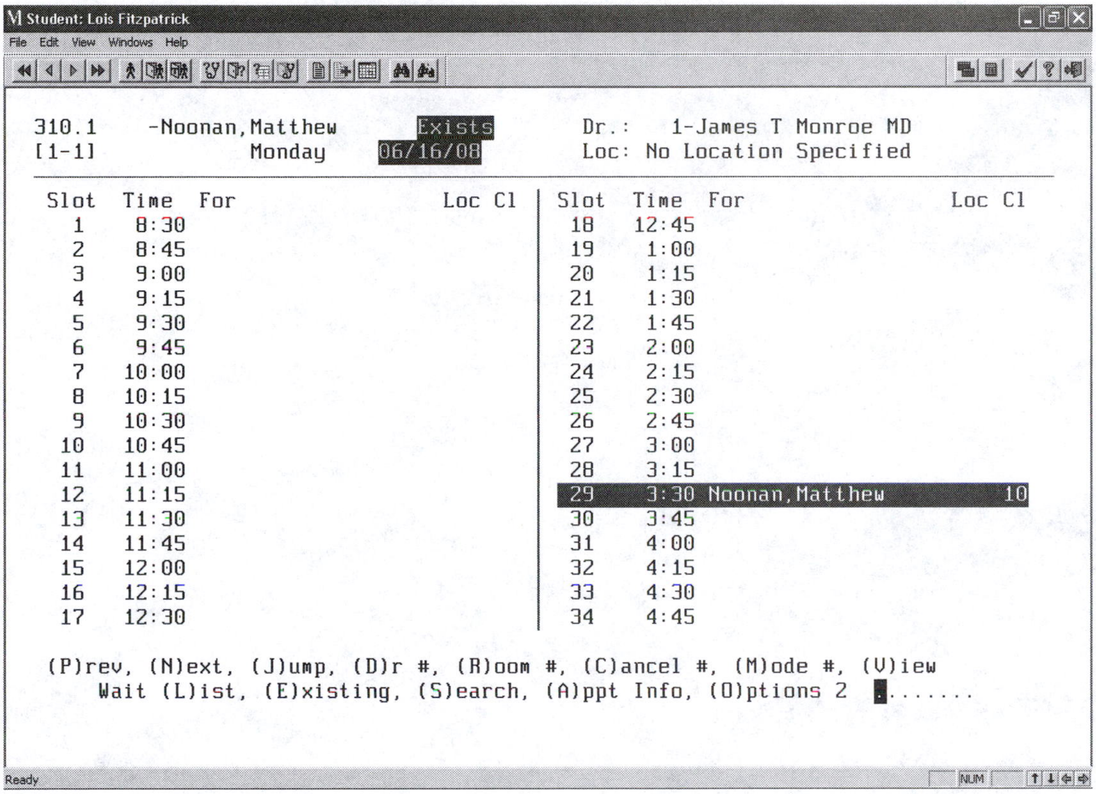

EXERCISE 7: DAILY LIST OF APPOINTMENTS

GOAL(S): Prepare an Appointments Detail Report by doctor.

1. Print an Appointments Detail Report by doctor, with remarks. Select only doctors 1-3 to print. Select the starting date as 06/02/2008 and ending date as 07/01/2008. Enter for all locations. Give your reports to your instructor.

EXERCISE 8: RESCHEDULE AN APPOINTMENT

CHRISTOPHER SALVANI

GOAL(S): Reschedule an appointment.

Christopher Salvani's appointment for a general check-up on April 24 at 2:30 with Dr. Simpson needs to be rescheduled for June 16.

1. Reschedule Christopher's general check-up appointment for 1:45 on June 16 with Dr. Simpson. Use CALLED as the reason code. Compare your screen to Figure 5-9.

Figure 5-9 Rescheduled Appointment

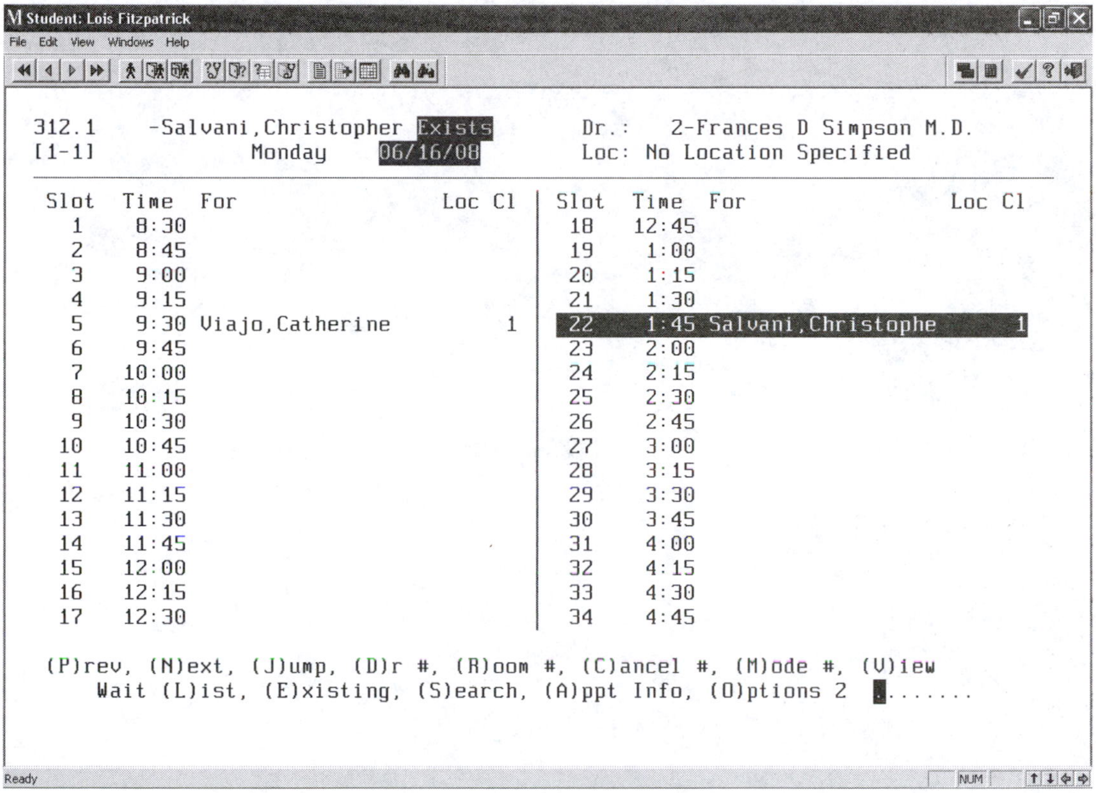

EXERCISE 9: RESCHEDULE WITH A DIFFERENT DOCTOR

DAVID FUENTAS

GOAL(S): Correct a scheduling error by rescheduling an appointment with a different doctor.

David Fuentas' personal consult appointment on June18 at 11:30 was entered on Dr. Carrington's schedule. Dr. Carrington is not available that day.

1. Using the information above, reschedule David's appointment for Dr. Monroe at 11:30 on June 18. Use NODOC for the reason code. Compare your screen to Figure 5-10.

Figure 5-10   Rescheduled – Fuentas

```
M Student: Lois Fitzpatrick                                          _ 🗗 ✕
File  Edit  View  Windows  Help

◀◀ ◀ ▶ ▶▶  🕴🗐🗐 🕑🗐🗐🗐  🗐🗐🗐  🗐🗐                        🗐🗐 ✓ ? 🗐

   314.1    -Fuentas,David      Exists      Dr.:  1-James T Monroe MD
   [1-3]                 Wednesday 06/18/08   Loc: No Location Specified
   ─────────────────────────────────────────────────────────────────
   Slot  Time  For            Loc Cl   Slot  Time  For           Loc Cl
    1    8:30                            18   12:45
    2    8:45                            19    1:00
    3    9:00                            20    1:15
    4    9:15                            21    1:30
    5    9:30                            22    1:45
    6    9:45                            23    2:00
    7   10:00                            24    2:15
    8   10:15                            25    2:30
    9   10:30                            26    2:45
   10   10:45                            27    3:00
   11   11:00                            28    3:15
   12   11:15                            29    3:30
   13   11:30 Fuentas,David        6     30    3:45
   14   11:45'Fuentas,David       6     31    4:00
   15   12:00                            32    4:15
   16   12:15                            33    4:30
   17   12:30                            34    4:45

   (P)rev, (N)ext, (J)ump, (D)r #, (R)oom #, (C)ancel #, (M)ode #, (V)iew
       Wait (L)ist, (E)xisting, (S)earch, (A)ppt Info, (O)ptions 2  ........

Ready                                                   NUM    ↑↓⇦⇨
```

EXERCISE 10: CANCELING AN APPOINTMENT

MARGARET MORGAN

GOAL(S): Cancel an appointment.

Margaret Morgan called to cancel a recheck appointment that is scheduled for June 17 with Dr. Carrington at 2:00.

1. Retrieve Margaret's account and cancel her appointment. Use CALL24 as the cancel code.

EXERCISE 11: POSTING PROCEDURES AND FOLLOW-UP APPOINTMENT

SONIA LOPEZ

GOAL(S): Post procedures and schedule an appointment.

1. Post the procedures from Sonia's encounter form using the information in Figure 5-11. Compare your screen to Figure 5-12.

Figure 5-11 Encounter Form – Lopez

Sydney Carrington & Associates P.A.
34 Sycamore Street Suite 300
Madison, CA 95653

Date: 06/02/2008

Voucher No.: 5001

Time:

Patient: Sonia Lopez
Guarantor:

Patient No: 317.0
Doctor: 2 – F. Simpson

CPT	DESCRIPTION	FEE
OFFICE/HOSPITAL CONSULTS		
☐ 99201	Office New:Focused Hx-Exam	
☐ 99202	Office New:Expanded Hx.Exam	
☐ 99211	Office Estb:Min./None Hx-Exa	
☐ 99212	Office Estb:Focused Hx-Exam	
☒ 99213	Office Estb:Expanded Hx-Exa	
☐ 99214	Office Estb:Detailed Hx-Exa	
☐ 99215	Office Estb:Comprhn Hx-Exam	
☐ 99221	Hosp. Initial:Comprh Hx-	
☐ 99223	Hosp. Ini:Comprh Hx-Exam/Hi	
☐ 99231	Hosp. Subsequent: S-Fwd	
☐ 99232	Hosp. Subsequent: Comprhn Hx	
☐ 99233	Hosp. Subsequent: Ex/Hi	
☐ 99238	Hospital Visit Discharge Ex	
☐ 99371	Telephone Consult - Simple	
☐ 99372	Telephone Consult - Intermed	
☐ 99373	Telephone Consult - Complex	
☐ 90840	Counseling - 25 minutes	
☐ 90806	Counseling - 50 minutes	
☐ 90865	Counseling - Special Interview	
IMMUNIZATIONS/INJECTIONS		
☐ 90585	BCG Vaccine	
☐ 90659	Influenza Virus Vaccine	
☐ 90701	Immunization-DTP	
☐ 90702	DT Vaccine	
☐ 90703	Tetanus Toxoids	
☐ 90732	Pneumococcal Vaccine	
☐ 90746	Hepatitis B Vaccine	
☐ 90749	Immunization: Unlisted	

CPT	DESCRIPTION	FEE
LABORATORY/RADIOLOGY		
☐ 81000	Urinalysis	
☐ 81002	Urinalysis; Pregnancy Test	
☐ 82951	Glucose Tolerance Test	
☐ 84478	Triglycerides	
☐ 84550	Uric Acid: Blood Chemistry	
☐ 84830	Ovulation Test	
☐ 85014	Hematocrit	
☒ 85032	Hemogram, Complete Blood Wk	
☐ 86403	Particle Agglutination Test	
☐ 86485	Skin Test; Candida	
☐ 86580	TB Intradermal Test	
☐ 86585	TB Tine Test	
☐ 87070	Culture	
☐ 70190	X-Ray; Optic Foramina	
☐ 70210	X-Ray Sinuses Complete	
☐ 71010	Radiological Exam Ent Spine	
☐ 71020	X-Ray Chest Pa & Lat	
☐ 72050	X-Ray Spine, Cerv (4 views)	
☐ 72090	X-Ray Spine; Scoliosis Ex	
☐ 72110	Spine, lumbosacral; a/p & Lat	
☐ 73030	Shoulder-Comp, min w/ 2vws	
☐ 73070	Elbow, anteropost & later vws	
☐ 73120	X-Ray; Hand, 2 views	
☐ 73560	X-Ray, Knee, 1 or 2 views	
☐ 74022	X-Ray; Abdomen, Complete	
☐ 75552	Cardiac Magnetic Res Img	
☐ 76020	X-Ray; Bone Age Studies	
☐ 77054	Mammary Ductogram Complete	
☐ 78465	Myocardial Perfusion Img	

CPT	DESCRIPTION	FEE
PROCEDURES/TESTS		
☐ 00452	Anesthesia for Rad Surgery	
☐ 11100	Skin Biopsy	
☐ 15852	Dressing Change	
☐ 29075	Cast Appl. - Lower Arm	
☐ 29530	Strapping of Knee	
☐ 29705	Removal/Revis of Cast w/Exa	
☐ 53670	Catheterization Incl. Suppl	
☐ 57452	Colposcopy	
☐ 57505	ECC	
☐ 69420	Myringotomy	
☐ 92081	Visual Field Examination	
☐ 92100	Serial Tonometry Exam	
☐ 92120	Tonography	
☐ 92552	Pure Tone Audiometry	
☐ 92567	Tympanometry	
☐ 93000	Electrocardiogram	
☐ 93015	Exercise Stress Test (ETT)	
☐ 93017	ETT Tracing Only	
☐ 93040	Electrocardiogram - Rhythm	
☐ 96100	Psychological Testing	
☐ 99000	Specimen Handling	
☐ 99058	Office Emergency Care	
☐ 99070	Surgical Tray - Misc.	
☐ 99080	Special Reports of Med Rec	
☐ 99195	Phlebotomy	
☐		
☐		
☐		

ICD-9 CODE DIAGNOSIS	
☐ 009.0	Infect. colitis, enteritis, & gastroenteritis
☐ 133.0	Scabies
☐ 174.9	Breast Cancer, Female, Unspecified
☐ 185	Malignant neoplasm of prostate
☐ 250.00	Diabetes Mellitus w/o mention of Complication
☐ 272.4	Hyperlipidemia
☐ 282.5	Anemia, Sickle-cell Trait
☐ 282.60	Sickle-cell disease, unspecified
☐ 285.9	Anemia, Unspecified
☐ 300.4	Dysthymic disorder
☐ 340	Multiple Sclerosis
☐ 342.90	Hemiplegia - Unspec.
☐ 346.90	Migraine, unspecified
☐ 352.9	Unspecified disorder of cranial nerves
☐ 354.0	Carpal Tunnel Syndrome
☐ 355.0	Sciatic Nerve Root Lesion
☐ 366.9	Cataract
☐ 386.00	Menier's disease, unspecified
☐ 401.1	Essential Hypertension, Benign
☐ 414.9	Ischemic Heart Disease
☐ 428.0	Congestive Heart Failure (CHF), unspecified

ICD-9 CODE DIAGNOSIS	
☐ 435.0	Basilar Artery Syndrome
☐ 440.0	Atherosclerosis
☐ 442.81	Carotid Artery
☐ 460	Common Cold (Acute Nasopharyngitis)
☐ 461.9	Acute Sinusitis
☐ 474.00	Chronic Tonsillitis & Adenoiditis
☐ 477.9	Allergic Rhinitis, Cause Unspecified
☐ 487.0	Influenza with pneumonia
☐ 496	Chronic Airway Obstruction
☐ 522.0	Pulpitis
☐ 524.60	Temporo-Mandibular Joint Disorder - Unspec.
☐ 536.8	Stomach Pain
☐ 553.3	Hiatal Hernia
☐ 564.1	Spastic Colon
☐ 574.40	Chronic Hepatitis, Unspecified
☐ 571.5	Cirrhosis of Liver w/o mention of alcohol
☐ 573.3	Hepatitis
☐ 575.2	Obstruction of Gallbladder
☐ 648.20	Anemia - Compl. Pregnancy
☐ 715.90	Osteoarthritis - Unspec.
☐ 721.3	Lumbar Osteo/Spondylarthrit

ICD-9 CODE DIAGNOSIS	
☐ 724.2	Pain: Lower Back
☐ 727.67	Rupture of Achilles Tendon
☐ 780.1	Hallucinations
☐ 780.3	Convulsions, Other
☐ 780.50	Sleep Disturbances, Unspecified
☐ 783.0	Anorexia
☐ 783.1	Abnormal Weight Gain
☒ 783.21	Abnormal Weight Loss
☐ 823.80	Fractured Tibia
☐ 823.81	Fractured Fibula
☐ 831.00	Dislocated Shoulder, Closed, Unspecified
☐ 835.00	Dislocated Hip, Closed, Unspecified
☐ 842.00	Sprained Wrist, Unspecified Site
☐ 845.00	Sprained Ankle, Unspecified Site
☐ 919.5	Insect Bite, Nonvenomous
☐ 921.1	Contus Eyelid/Perioc Area
☐ v16.3	Fam. Hist of Breast Cancer
☐ v17.4	Fam. Hist of Cardiovasc Dis
☐ v20.2	Well Child
☐ v22.0	Pregnancy - First Normal
☐ v22.1	Pregnancy - Normal

Previous Balance	Today's Charges	Total Due	Amount Paid	New Balance
_____	_____	_____	_____	_____

Follow Up

PRN _____ Weeks _____ Months _____ Units _____

Next Appointment Date: June. 23   Time: 10:45   Recheck

I hereby authorize release of any information acquired in the course of examination or treatment and allow a photocopy of my signature to be used.

Figure 5-12   Two Procedures Posted

```
M Student: Lois Fitzpatrick                                              _ ☐ ☒
File  Edit  View  Windows  Help

 Patient #: 317.0    [Sonia Lopez              ]        Dept.    : 0
 Voucher #: 5001         Doctor # :  2 Simpson M.D., Fran  Location :
                         Supervisor:  2 Simpson M.D., Fran
 Dates    P.O.S.  Procedure   Modifier Diag. 1-4    Units      Charges   T.O.S.

 06/02/08  3     ..........                      .....  $    15.00  1

 |Blood Count, Manual Cell Count    |783.21     Abnormal Weight Loss
 Comment:                           |
                                    |  .........
                                    |  .........
 Ins: Primary#: 7.0       Assign: Y    Secondary#: 0.0       EMC Billable: Y
 [Posted]──────────────────────────────────────────────────────────────
        Date     Co #  Dr# Procedure   Diag      Units    Charges  Total Chgs

   1  06/02/08 7   2  99213     783.21    1.00    40.00    40.00
   2  06/02/08 7   2  85032     783.21    1.00    15.00    55.00




 Enter '?', '↑', '?code' for Help, '?~' for Macros, or '%' for Standing Orders

Ready                                                    NUM   ↑↓←→
```

2. Schedule Sonia's next appointment as indicated on her encounter form. Compare your screen to Figure 5-13.

Figure 5-13   Follow-up Appointment – Lopez

```
M Student: Lois Fitzpatrick                                              _ ☐ ☒
File  Edit  View  Windows  Help

 317.0    -Lopez,Sonia    Exists     Dr.:   2-Frances D Simpson M.D.
 [1-1]          Monday    06/23/08   Loc: No Location Specified

 Slot  Time  For            Loc Cl   Slot  Time  For            Loc Cl
   1   8:30                            18   12:45
   2   8:45                            19   1:00
   3   9:00                            20   1:15
   4   9:15                            21   1:30
   5   9:30                            22   1:45
   6   9:45                            23   2:00
   7   10:00                           24   2:15
   8   10:15                           25   2:30
   9   10:30                           26   2:45
  10   10:45 Lopez,Sonia        5      27   3:00
  11   11:00                           28   3:15
  12   11:15                           29   3:30
  13   11:30                           30   3:45
  14   11:45                           31   4:00
  15   12:00                           32   4:15
  16   12:15                           33   4:30
  17   12:30                           34   4:45

 (P)rev, (N)ext, (J)ump, (D)r #, (R)oom #, (C)ancel #, (M)ode #, (V)iew
    Wait (L)ist, (E)xisting, (S)earch, (A)ppt Info, (O)ptions 2 ........

Ready                                                    NUM   ↑↓←→
```

EXERCISE 12: POST PROCEDURES AND MULTI-SLOT FOLLOW-UP APPOINTMENT

GARY BRINKMAN

GOAL(S): Post procedures and schedule an appointment for a multiple slot.

1. Post three procedures from Gary's encounter form. Compare your screen to Figure 5-15.

Figure 5-14 Encounter Form – Brinkman

Sydney Carrington & Associates P.A.
34 Sycamore Street Suite 300
Madison, CA 95653

Date: 06/02/2008   Voucher No.: 5002

Time:

Patient: Gary Brinkman   Patient No: 318.0
Guarantor: Doctor: 1 – J. Monroe

CPT	DESCRIPTION	FEE	CPT	DESCRIPTION	FEE	CPT	DESCRIPTION	FEE
OFFICE/HOSPITAL CONSULTS			**LABORATORY/RADIOLOGY**			**PROCEDURES/TESTS**		
99201	Office New:Focused Hx Exam		81000	Urinalysis		00162	Anesthesia for Rad Surgery	
99202	Office New:Expanded Hx.Exam		81002	Urinalysis; Pregnancy Test		11100	Skin Biopsy	
99211	Office Estb:Min./None Hx-Exa		82951	Glucose Tolerance Test		15852	Dressing Change	
99212	Office Estb:Focused Hx-Exam		84478	Triglycerides		29075	Cast Appl. - Lower Arm	
99213	Office Estb:Expanded Hx-Exa		84550	Uric Acid: Blood Chemistry		29530	Strapping of Knee	
99214	Office Estb:Detailed Hx-Exa		84830	Ovulation Test		29705	Removal/Revis of Cast w/Exa	
99215	Office Estb:Comprhn Hx-Exam		85014	Hematocrit		53670	Catheterization Incl. Suppl	
99221	Hosp. Initial:Comprh Hx-		85032	Hemogram, Complete Blood Wk		57452	Colposcopy	
99223	Hosp. Ini:Comprh Hx-Exam/Hi		86403	Particle Agglutination Test		57505	ECC	
99231	Hosp. Subsequent: S-Fwd		86485	Skin Test; Candida		69420	Myringotomy	
99232	Hosp. Subsequent: Comprhn Hx		86580	TB Intradermal Test		92081	Visual Field Examination	
99233	Hosp. Subsequent: Ex/Hi		86585	TB Tine Test		92100	Serial Tonometry Exam	
99238	Hospital Visit Discharge Ex		87070	Culture		92120	Tonography	
99371	Telephone Consult - Simple		70190	X-Ray; Optic Foramina		92552	Pure Tone Audiometry	
99372	Telephone Consult - Intermed		70210	X-Ray Sinuses Complete		92567	Tympanometry	
99373	Telephone Consult - Complex		71010	Radiological Exam Ent Spine		93000	Electrocardiogram	
90840	Counseling - 25 minutes		71020	X-Ray Chest Pa & Lat		93015	Exercise Stress Test (ETT)	
90806	Counseling - 50 minutes		72050	X-Ray Spine, Cerv (4 views)		93017	ETT Tracing Only	
90865	Counseling - Special Interview		72090	X-Ray Spine; Scoliosis Ex		93040	Electrocardiogram - Rhythm	
			72110	Spine, lumbosacral; a/p & Lat		96100	Psychological Testing	
IMMUNIZATIONS/INJECTIONS			73030	Shoulder-Comp, min w/ 2vws		99000	Specimen Handling	
90585	BCG Vaccine		73070	Elbow, anteropost & later vws		99058	Office Emergency Care	
90659	Influenza Virus Vaccine		73120	X-Ray; Hand, 2 views		99070	Surgical Tray - Misc.	
90701	Immunization-DTP		73560	X-Ray, Knee, 1 or 2 views		99080	Special Reports of Med Rec	
90702	DT Vaccine		74022	X-Ray; Abdomen, Complete		99195	Phlebotomy	
90703	Tetanus Toxoids		75552	Cardiac Magnetic Res Img				
90732	Pneumococcal Vaccine		76020	X-Ray; Bone Age Studies				
90746	Hepatitis B Vaccine		77054	Mammary Ductogram Complete				
90749	Immunization: Unlisted		78465	Myocardial Perfusion Img				

ICD-9 CODE DIAGNOSIS			ICD-9 CODE DIAGNOSIS			ICD-9 CODE DIAGNOSIS		
009.0	Infect. colitis, enteritis, & gastroenteritis		435.0	Basilar Artery Syndrome		724.2	Pain: Lower Back	
133.0	Scabies		440.0	Atherosclerosis		727.67	Rupture of Achilles Tendon	
174.9	Breast Cancer, Female, Unspecified		442.81	Carotid Artery		780.1	Hallucinations	
185	Malignant neoplasm of prostate		460	Common Cold (Acute Nasopharyngitis)		780.3	Convulsions, Other	
250.00	Diabetes Mellitus w/o mention of Complication		461.9	Acute Sinusitis		780.50	Sleep Disturbances, Unspecified	
272.4	Hyperlipidemia		474.00	Chronic Tonsillitis & Adenoiditis		783.0	Anorexia	
282.5	Anemia, Sickle-cell Trait		477.9	Allergic Rhinitis, Cause Unspecified		783.1	Abnormal Weight Gain	
282.60	Sickle-cell disease, unspecified		487.0	Influenza with pneumonia		783.21	Abnormal Weight Loss	
285.9	Anemia, Unspecified		496	Chronic Airway Obstruction		823.80	Fractured Tibia	
300.4	Dysthymic disorder		522.0	Pulpitis		823.81	Fractured Fibula	
340	Multiple Sclerosis		524.60	Temporo-Mandibular Joint Disorder - Unspec.		831.00	Dislocated Shoulder, Closed, Unspecified	
342.90	Hemiplegia - Unspec.		536.8	Stomach Pain		835.00	Dislocated Hip, Closed, Unspecified	
346.90	Migraine, unspecified		553.3	Hiatal Hernia		842.00	Sprained Wrist, Unspecified Site	
352.9	Unspecified disorder of cranial nerves		564.1	Spastic Colon		845.00	Sprained Ankle, Unspecified Site	
354.0	Carpal Tunnel Syndrome		574.40	Chronic Hepatitis, Unspecified		919.5	Insect Bite, Nonvenomous	
355.0	Sciatic Nerve Root Lesion		571.5	Cirrhosis of Liver w/o mention of alcohol		921.1	Contus Eyelid/Perioc Area	
366.9	Cataract		573.3	Hepatitis		v16.3	Fam. Hist of Breast Cancer	
386.00	Menier's disease, unspecified		575.2	Obstruction of Gallbladder		v17.4	Fam. Hist of Cardiovasc Dis	
401.1	Essential Hypertension, Benign		648.20	Anemia - Compl. Pregnancy		v20.2	Well Child	
414.9	Ischemic Heart Disease		715.90	Osteoarthritis - Unspec.		v22.0	Pregnancy - First Normal	
428.0	Congestive Heart Failure (CHF), unspecified		721.3	Lumbar Osteo/Spondylarthrit		v22.1	Pregnancy - Normal	

Previous Balance	Today's Charges	Total Due	Amount Paid	New Balance

Follow Up

PRN _____ Weeks _____ Months _____ Units _____

Next Appointment Date: June 4   Time: 03:15   Personal consult; 30 minutes

I hereby authorize release of any information acquired in the course of examination or treatment and allow a photocopy of my signature to be used.

2. Schedule Gary's next appointment as indicated on his encounter form. Compare your screen to Figure 5-16.

Figure 5-15   Three Procedures Posted – Brinkman

```
 M Student: Lois Fitzpatrick                                                    _ 🗗 ✕
 File  Edit  View  Windows  Help

 🔲🕊🕊 ⏱🔲🐾🕊💲 🖊🔲🔲🔲 🔲🔲 🔲🔲 🔲🔲🔲🔲                          🔲🔲 ✓?🔲

   Patient #: 318.0     [Gary Brinkman                    ]      Dept.   :  0
   Voucher #: 5002              Doctor #  :   1 Monroe MD, James   Location :
                                Supervisor:   1 Monroe MD, James
   Dates     P.O.S.   Procedure   Modifier Diag. 1-4    Units       Charges   T.O.S.

   06/02/08   3    ...........                          ....   $    40.00   1

   |Glucose Tolerance Test           |250.00     Diabetes Mellitus w/o mention |
   Comment:                          |
                                     | ..........
                                     | ..........
   Ins: Primary#: 5.0       Assign: Y     Secondary#: 0.0      EMC Billable: Y
   [Posted]─────────────────────────────────────────────────────────────────
         Date    Co #  Dr# Procedure   Diag      Units      Charges   Total Chgs

     1  06/02/08 5     1   99214    250.00       1.00       50.00      50.00
     2  06/02/08 5     1   81000    250.00       1.00        8.00      58.00
     3  06/02/08 5     1   82951    250.00       1.00       40.00      98.00




        Enter '?', '!', '?code' for Help, '?~' for Macros, or '%' for Standing Orders


 Ready                                                                  NUM   ↑↓←→
```

Figure 5-16   Return Appointment – Brinkman

```
 M Student: Lois Fitzpatrick                                                    _ 🗗 ✕
 File  Edit  View  Windows  Help

 ⏮◀▶⏭ 🕊🔲🔲 🔲🔲🔲🔲 🔲🔲🔲 🔲🔲                                    🔲🔲 ✓?🔲

   318.0     -Brinkman,Gary      Exists      Dr.:   1-James T Monroe MD
   [1-3]                 Wednesday 06/04/08    Loc: No Location Specified

   Slot  Time  For              Loc Cl  │ Slot  Time  For              Loc Cl
    1    8:30                            │  18   12:45
    2    8:45                            │  19   1:00
    3    9:00                            │  20   1:15
    4    9:15                            │  21   1:30
    5    9:30                            │  22   1:45
    6    9:45                            │  23   2:00
    7   10:00                            │  24   2:15
    8   10:15                            │  25   2:30
    9   10:30                            │  26   2:45
   10   10:45                            │  27   3:00
   11   11:00                            │  28   3:15 Brinkman,Gary        6
   12   11:15                            │  29   3:30'Brinkman,Gary        6
   13   11:30                            │  30   3:45
   14   11:45                            │  31   4:00
   15   12:00                            │  32   4:15
   16   12:15                            │  33   4:30
   17   12:30                            │  34   4:45

   (P)rev, (N)ext, (J)ump, (D)r #, (R)oom #, (C)ancel #, (M)ode #, (V)iew
        Wait (L)ist, (E)xisting, (S)earch, (A)ppt Info, (O)ptions 2 ▮.......


 Ready                                                                  NUM   ↑↓←→
```

EXERCISE 13: CANCEL AN APPOINTMENT AND ADD HOSPITAL ROUNDS

GARY BRINKMAN

GOAL(S): In this exercise, you will cancel an existing appointment, add a patient to a hospital rounds report, and print the report.

Gary Brinkman calls the office later the same day, following his last appointment (Exercise 12). Dr. Monroe is going to admit Gary Brinkman to Jefferson Memorial Hospital due to his diabetic condition. He is expected to be in the hospital for three days. Use the information provided to create the report.

1. Cancel Gary's existing appointment on June 4.

2. Add Gary to hospital rounds to have this entry appear on Dr. Monroe's rounds report.

3. Gary's hospital ID # is 157239630.

4. Gary's admission is urgent. Compare your screen to Figure 5-17.

5. Print a hospital rounds report sorted by doctor, including tomorrow's admissions, for all doctors and facilities. Give your report to your instructor.

Figure 5-17   Hospital Admission

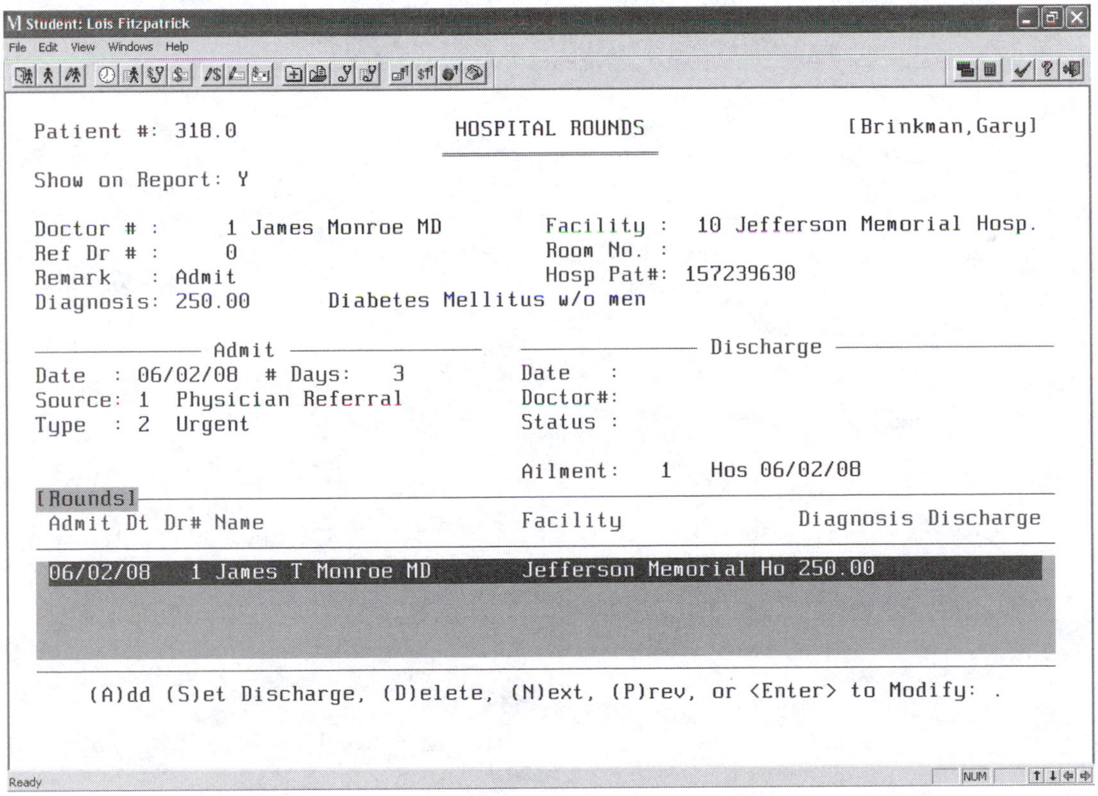

EXERCISE 14: POST PROCEDURE CODES FOR HOSPITAL VISITS

GOAL(S): In this exercise you will need to use the procedure code help window to locate codes.

Dr. Monroe has discharged Gary Brinkman from Jefferson Memorial Hospital after his four-day stay. Using the Hospital Rounds report (Figure 5-18) and the information provided below, post the charges to his account.

Figure 5-18   Hospital Rounds Report

```
M Student: Lois Fitzpatrick                                                    _ |□|X
File  Edit  View  Windows  Help

06/02/08            HOSPITAL ROUNDS REPORT BY SERVICE FACILITY        Page    1
                            (1)James T Monroe MD
                        (10)Jefferson Memorial Hosp.

    Patient/Diagnosis/Admit        Pat #        Room/Comment        Ref Dr/Hosp ID

    Brinkman,Gary                  318.0
      Diabetes Mellitus w/o mention of Complic  Admit              157239630
      Date:06/02/08 Source:Physician Referral   Type:Urgent


                        Discharge to home 06/05/08




Ready                                                          NUM      ↑↓⇔⇒
```

Become familiar with the hospital rounds report and answer the following questions before attempting the data entry:

1. What is the date of admission for Gary Brinkman?

2. What is the date of discharge for Gary Brinkman?

3. Which doctor cared for Gary Brinkman during his hospital stay?

Gary Brinkman's hospitalization charges will include:

06/02/2008	One Procedure: Admission History and Comprehensive Physical Exam (Hospital Initial: Comprh Hx-Exam/Hi)
06/03/2008, 06/04/2008	Two Procedures: Hospital Visit Expanded (Hosp. Subsequent: Comprh Hx-Exam/Mod)
06/05/2008	One Procedure: Hospital Discharge Exam (Hospital Visit Discharge Exam)

When you have posted the hospital visits listed above, compare your screen to Figure 5-19.

Figure 5-19   Posted – Three Hospital Visits

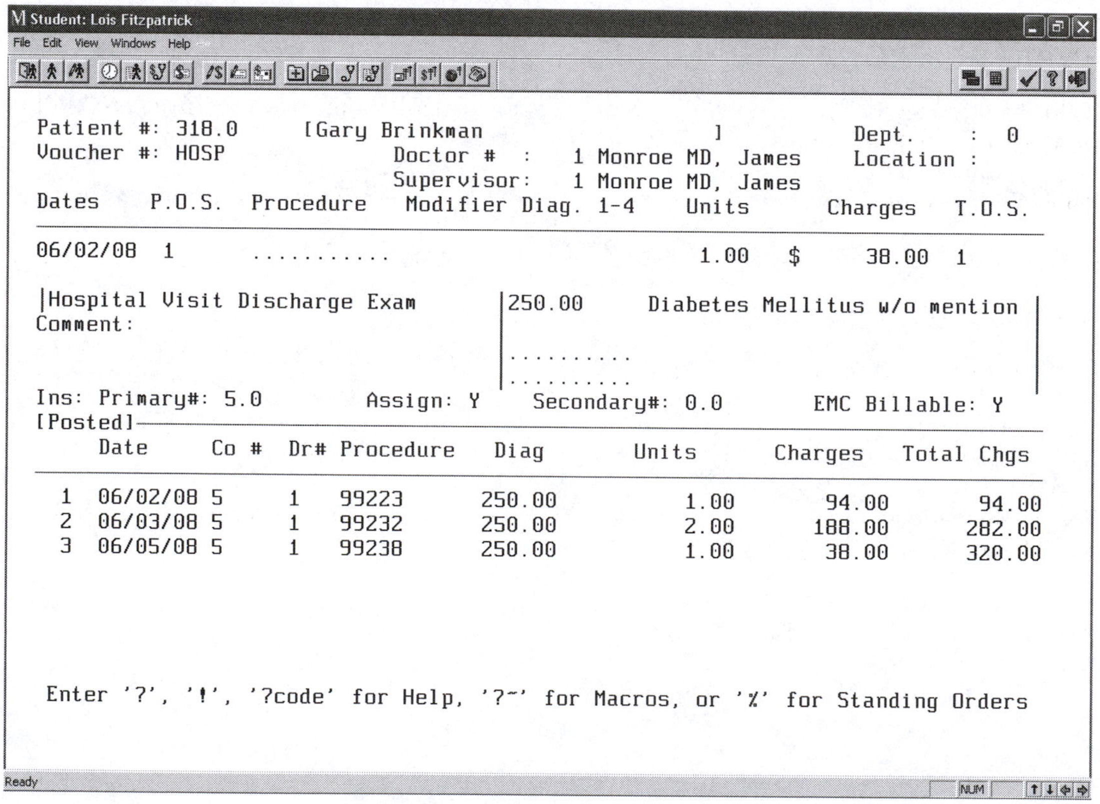

U N I T 6

Practice Management

In the unit exercises that follow, you will post procedures, post patient payments, post negative adjustments, transfer payment responsibility, use automatic crediting, and post insurance payments.

EXERCISE 1: POST PROCEDURES AND PATIENT PAYMENT

WAYNE MILES; ACCOUNT 319

GOAL(S): In this exercise, you will post procedures and payments from the Procedure Entry screen for Wayne Miles, who will pay in full for the visit.

1. Before posting your entry, study the encounter form in Figure 6-1. Answer the following questions.

   a. How many procedures were performed? _____

   b. What is the diagnosis? _____

   c. What is the total charge for this visit? _____

2. Based on the information found on the encounter form, post the charges for Wayne Miles. When you have correctly posted all three procedures, compare your screen to Figure 6-2.

3. Wayne Miles provides a check for the full amount of the visit. See Figure 6-3. Apply the check for $123 to his account. Compare your screen to Figure 6-4.

Figure 6-1 Encounter Form – Miles

Sydney Carrington & Associates P.A.
34 Sycamore Street Suite 300
Madison, CA 95653

Date: 06/02/2008

Voucher No.: 1163

Time:

Patient: Wayne Miles
Guarantor:

Patient No: 319.0
Doctor: 2 – F. Simpson

□ CPT	DESCRIPTION	FEE
OFFICE/HOSPITAL CONSULTS		
□ 99201	Office New:Focused Hx-Exam	
□ 99202	Office New:Expanded Hx.Exam	
□ 99211	Office Estb:Min./None Hx-Exa	
□ 99212	Office Estb:Focused Hx-Exam	
□ 99213	Office Estb:Expanded Hx-Exa	
☒ 99214	Office Estb:Detailed Hx-Exa	$50
□ 99215	Office Estb:Comprhn Hx-Exam	
□ 99221	Hosp. Initial:Comprh Hx-	
□ 99223	Hosp. Ini:Comprh Hx-Exam/Hi	
□ 99231	Hosp. Subsequent: S-Fwd	
□ 99232	Hosp. Subsequent: Comprhn Hx	
□ 99233	Hosp. Subsequent: Ex/Hi	
□ 99238	Hospital Visit Discharge Ex	
□ 99371	Telephone Consult - Simple	
□ 99372	Telephone Consult - Intermed	
□ 99373	Telephone Consult - Complex	
□ 90840	Counseling - 25 minutes	
□ 90806	Counseling - 50 minutes	
□ 90865	Counseling - Special Interview	
IMMUNIZATIONS/INJECTIONS		
□ 90585	BCG Vaccine	
□ 90659	Influenza Virus Vaccine	
□ 90701	Immunization-DTP	
□ 90702	DT Vaccine	
□ 90703	Tetanus Toxoids	
□ 90732	Pneumococcal Vaccine	
□ 90746	Hepatitis B Vaccine	
□ 90749	Immunization: Unlisted	

□ CPT	DESCRIPTION	FEE
LABORATORY/RADIOLOGY		
□ 81000	Urinalysis	
□ 81002	Urinalysis; Pregnancy Test	
□ 82951	Glucose Tolerance Test	
□ 84478	Triglycerides	
□ 84550	Uric Acid: Blood Chemistry	
□ 84830	Ovulation Test	
□ 85014	Hematocrit	
☒ 85032	Hemogram, Complete Blood Wk	$15
□ 86403	Particle Agglutination Test	
□ 86485	Skin Test; Candida	
□ 86580	TB Intradermal Test	
□ 86585	TB Tine Test	
□ 87070	Culture	
□ 70190	X-Ray; Optic Foramina	
□ 70210	X-Ray Sinuses Complete	
□ 71010	Radiological Exam Ent Spine	
☒ 71020	X-Ray Chest Pa & Lat	$58
□ 72050	X-Ray Spine, Cerv (4 views)	
□ 72090	X-Ray Spine; Scoliosis Ex	
□ 72110	Spine, lumbosacral; a/p & Lat	
□ 73030	Shoulder-Comp, min w/ 2vws	
□ 73070	Elbow, anteropost & later vws	
□ 73120	X-Ray; Hand, 2 views	
□ 73560	X-Ray, Knee, 1 or 2 views	
□ 74022	X-Ray; Abdomen, Complete	
□ 75552	Cardiac Magnetic Res Img	
□ 76020	X-Ray; Bone Age Studies	
□ 77054	Mammary Ductogram Complete	
□ 78465	Myocardial Perfusion Img	

□ CPT	DESCRIPTION	FEE
PROCEDURES/TESTS		
□ 00452	Anesthesia for Rad Surgery	
□ 11100	Skin Biopsy	
□ 15852	Dressing Change	
□ 29075	Cast Appl. - Lower Arm	
□ 29530	Strapping of Knee	
□ 29705	Removal/Revis of Cast w/Exa	
□ 53670	Catheterization Incl. Suppl	
□ 57452	Colposcopy	
□ 57505	ECC	
□ 69420	Myringotomy	
□ 92081	Visual Field Examination	
□ 92100	Serial Tonometry Exam	
□ 92120	Tonography	
□ 92552	Pure Tone Audiometry	
□ 92567	Tympanometry	
□ 93000	Electrocardiogram	
□ 93015	Exercise Stress Test (ETT)	
□ 93017	ETT Tracing Only	
□ 93040	Electrocardiogram - Rhythm	
□ 96100	Psychological Testing	
□ 99000	Specimen Handling	
□ 99058	Office Emergency Care	
□ 99070	Surgical Tray - Misc.	
□ 99080	Special Reports of Med Rec	
□ 99195	Phlebotomy	
□ _____	_____	
□ _____	_____	
□ _____	_____	
□ _____	_____	

□	**ICD-9 CODE DIAGNOSIS**
□ 009.0	Infect. colitis, enteritis, & gastroenteritis
□ 133.0	Scabies
□ 174.9	Breast Cancer, Female, Unspecified
□ 185	Malignant neoplasm of prostate
□ 250.00	Diabetes Mellitus w/o mention of Complication
□ 272.4	Hyperlipidemia
□ 282.5	Anemia, Sickle-cell Trait
□ 282.60	Sickle-cell disease, unspecified
□ 285.9	Anemia, Unspecified
□ 300.4	Dysthymic disorder
□ 340	Multiple Sclerosis
□ 342.90	Hemiplegia - Unspec.
□ 346.90	Migraine, unspecified
□ 352.9	Unspecified disorder of cranial nerves
□ 354.0	Carpal Tunnel Syndrome
□ 355.0	Sclatic Nerve Root Lesion
□ 366.9	Cataract
□ 386.00	Menier's disease, unspecified
□ 401.1	Essential Hypertension, Benign
□ 414.9	Ischemic Heart Disease
□ 428.0	Congestive Heart Failure (CHF), unspecified

□	**ICD-9 CODE DIAGNOSIS**
□ 435.0	Basilar Artery Syndrome
□ 440.0	Atherosclerosis
□ 442.81	Carotid Artery
□ 460	Common Cold (Acute Nasopharyngitis)
□ 461.9	Acute Sinusitis
□ 474.00	Chronic Tonsillitis & Adenoiditis
□ 477.9	Allergic Rhinitis, Cause Unspecified
□ 487.0	Influenza with pneumonia
□ 496	Chronic Airway Obstruction
□ 522.0	Pulpitis
□ 524.60	Temporo-Mandibular Joint Disorder - Unspec.
□ 536.8	Stomach Pain
□ 553.3	Hiatal Hernia
□ 564.1	Spastic Colon
□ 574.40	Chronic Hepatitis, Unspecified
□ 571.5	Cirrhosis of Liver w/o mention of alcohol
□ 573.3	Hepatitis
□ 575.2	Obstruction of Gallbladder
□ 648.20	Anemia - Compl. Pregnancy
□ 715.90	Osteoarthritis - Unspec.
□ 721.3	Lumbar Osteo/Spondylarthrit

□	**ICD-9 CODE DIAGNOSIS**
□ 724.2	Pain: Lower Back
□ 727.67	Rupture of Achilles Tendon
□ 780.1	Hallucinations
□ 780.3	Convulsions, Other
□ 780.50	Sleep Disturbances, Unspecified
□ 783.0	Anorexia
□ 783.1	Abnormal Weight Gain
□ 783.21	Abnormal Weight Loss
□ 823.80	Fractured Tibia
□ 823.81	Fractured Fibula
□ 831.00	Dislocated Shoulder, Closed, Unspecified
□ 835.00	Dislocated Hip, Closed, Unspecified
□ 842.00	Sprained Wrist, Unspecified Site
□ 845.00	Sprained Ankle, Unspecified Site
□ 919.5	Insect Bite, Nonvenomous
□ 921.1	Contus Eyelid/Perioc Area
□ v16.3	Fam. Hist of Breast Cancer
□ v17.4	Fam. Hist of Cardiovasc Dis
□ v20.2	Well Child
□ v22.0	Pregnancy - First Normal
□ v22.1	Pregnancy - Normal
X 480.0	Viral Pneumonia

Previous Balance	Today's Charges	Total Due	Amount Paid	New Balance
_____	_____	_____	$123 check #1624	

Follow Up

PRN _____ Weeks _____   Months _____ Units _____

Next Appointment Date: Time:

I hereby authorize release of any information acquired in the course of
examination or treatment and allow a photocopy of my signature to be used.

_____   _____

Figure 6-2 Three Procedures Posted – Miles

```
M Student: Lois Fitzpatrick                                                    _ 🗗 ⊠
File  Edit  View  Windows  Help
┌─────────────────────────────────────────────────────────────────────────────┐
│                                                                               │
│    Patient #: 319.0    [Wayne Miles                    ]      Dept.   :  0    │
│    Voucher #: 1163                Doctor # :   2 Simpson M.D., Fran Location : │
│                                   Supervisor:  2 Simpson M.D., Fran           │
│    Dates    P.O.S.   Procedure   Modifier Diag. 1-4   Units    Charges  T.O.S.│
│                                                                               │
│    06/02/08  3      ▮..........                       ....  $     58.00  1    │
│    |X-Ray Chest Pa & Lat               |480.0    Viral Pneumonia due to adenovi│
│    Comment:                            |                                      │
│                                        |.........                            │
│                                        |.........                            │
│    Ins: Primary#: 0.0      Assign: .    Secondary#: .......  EMC Billable: .  │
│    [Posted]─────────────────────────────────────────────────────────────────│
│         Date      Co #  Dr# Procedure  Diag     Units    Charges  Total Chgs  │
│        ───────────────────────────────────────────────────────────────────── │
│      1  06/02/08   2    99214      480.0        1.00     50.00     50.00       │
│      2  06/02/08   2    85032      480.0        1.00     15.00     65.00       │
│      3  06/02/08   2    71020      480.0        1.00     58.00    123.00       │
│                                                                               │
│                                                                               │
│                                                                               │
│     Enter '?', '!', '?code' for Help, '?~' for Macros, or '%' for Standing Orders│
│                                                                               │
└───────────────────────────────────────────────────────────────────────────────┘
Ready                                                          NUM      ↑↓⇐⇒
```

Figure 6-3 Check from Patient – Miles

```
┌─────────────────────────────────────────────────────────────────────────────┐
│                                                                               │
│   Wayne and Sheila Miles                                          1624        │
│   40 Kentucky Lane                                                            │
│   Madison, CA 95653-0235                 June 2           2008                │
│                                                                               │
│   Pay to the                                                                  │
│   order of      Sydney Carrington & Associates          $  123.00            │
│                                                                               │
│         One hundred twenty three and 00/100                      Dollars      │
│                                                                               │
│   FIRST COMMUNITY BANK                                                        │
│   Madison, California                                                         │
│                                                                               │
│   Memo                                        Wayne Miles                     │
│                                                                               │
│   ⑆O42O43392⑆  34274⑈  1624                                                   │
│                                                                               │
└───────────────────────────────────────────────────────────────────────────────┘
```

Figure 6-4 Payment from Patient

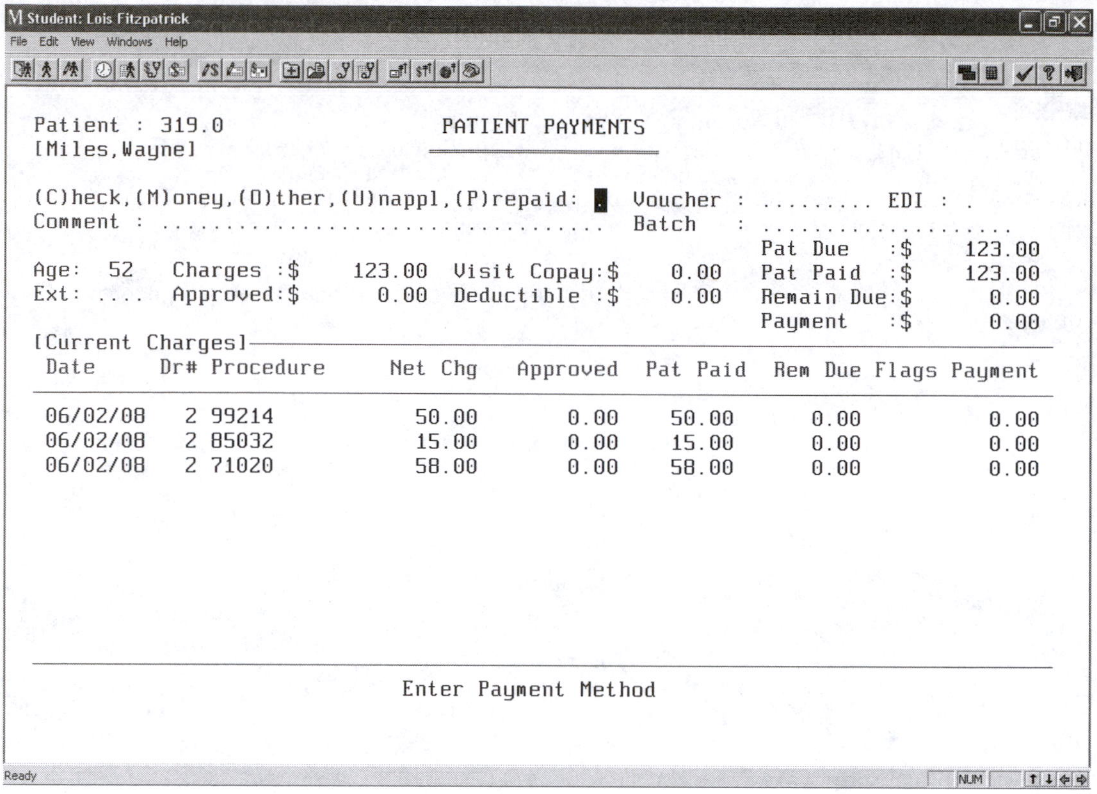

```
M Student: Lois Fitzpatrick                                          _ ⊡ X
File  Edit  View  Windows  Help
[toolbar icons]                                                    [icons]

  Patient : 319.0                    PATIENT PAYMENTS
  [Miles,Wayne]
  _____

  (C)heck,(M)oney,(O)ther,(U)nappl,(P)repaid: ▮  Voucher : ........ EDI : .
  Comment : ................................    Batch   : ..................
                                                       Pat Due   :$    123.00
  Age:  52    Charges :$    123.00  Visit Copay:$  0.00  Pat Paid  :$    123.00
  Ext: ....   Approved:$      0.00  Deductible :$  0.00  Remain Due:$      0.00
                                                       Payment   :$      0.00
  [Current Charges]──────────────────────────────────────────────────────────
   Date      Dr# Procedure     Net Chg   Approved   Pat Paid   Rem Due Flags Payment

   06/02/08   2 99214           50.00      0.00       50.00      0.00          0.00
   06/02/08   2 85032           15.00      0.00       15.00      0.00          0.00
   06/02/08   2 71020           58.00      0.00       58.00      0.00          0.00




  _____

                        Enter Payment Method


Ready                                                        NUM    ↑↓←→
```

EXERCISE 2: PATIENT COPAYMENT

LEANNA RAMIREZ; ACCOUNT 320

GOAL(S): In this exercise, you will post procedures and a payment from the Procedure Entry screen for Leanna Ramirez, who will pay a $10 copayment.

1. Before posting your entry, study the encounter form in Figure 6-5. Note the charges and diagnosis before attempting the data entry.

2. Based on the information found on the encounter form, post the charges for Leanna Ramirez. Compare your screen to Figure 6-6.

3. Leanna Ramirez provides a check for her $10 copayment. See Figure 6-7. Apply the check for $10 to her account. Compare your screen to Figure 6-8.

Figure 6-5 Encounter Form – Ramirez

Sydney Carrington & Associates P.A.
34 Sycamore Street Suite 300
Madison, CA 95653

Date: 06/02/2008   Voucher No.: 1344

Time:

Patient: Leanna Ramirez   Patient No: 320.0
Guarantor: Doctor: 2 - J. Monroe

☐ CPT	DESCRIPTION	FEE
OFFICE/HOSPITAL CONSULTS		
☐ 99201	Office New:Focused Hx-Exam	
☐ 99202	Office New:Expanded Hx.Exam	
☐ 99211	Office Estb:Min./None Hx-Exa	
☐ 99212	Office Estb:Focused Hx-Exam	
☒ 99213	Office Estb:Expanded Hx-Exa	$40
☐ 99214	Office Estb:Detailed Hx-Exa	
☐ 99215	Office Estb:Comprhn Hx-Exam	
☐ 99221	Hosp. Initial:Comprh Hx-	
☐ 99223	Hosp. Ini:Comprh Hx-Exam/Hi	
☐ 99231	Hosp. Subsequent: S-Fwd	
☐ 99232	Hosp. Subsequent: Comprhn Hx	
☐ 99233	Hosp. Subsequent: Ex/Hi	
☐ 99238	Hospital Visit Discharge Ex	
☐ 99371	Telephone Consult - Simple	
☐ 99372	Telephone Consult - Intermed	
☐ 99373	Telephone Consult - Complex	
☐ 90840	Counseling - 25 minutes	
☐ 90806	Counseling - 50 minutes	
☐ 90865	Counseling - Special Interview	
IMMUNIZATIONS/INJECTIONS		
☐ 90585	BCG Vaccine	
☐ 90659	Influenza Virus Vaccine	
☐ 90701	Immunization-DTP	
☐ 90702	DT Vaccine	
☐ 90703	Tetanus Toxoids	
☐ 90732	Pneumococcal Vaccine	
☐ 90746	Hepatitis B Vaccine	
☐ 90749	Immunization: Unlisted	

☐ CPT	DESCRIPTION	FEE
LABORATORY/RADIOLOGY		
☐ 81000	Urinalysis	
☐ 81002	Urinalysis; Pregnancy Test	
☐ 82951	Glucose Tolerance Test	
☐ 84478	Triglycerides	
☐ 84550	Uric Acid: Blood Chemistry	
☐ 84830	Ovulation Test	
☐ 85014	Hematocrit	
☒ 85032	Hemogram, Complete Blood Wk	$15
☐ 86403	Particle Agglutination Test	
☐ 86485	Skin Test; Candida	
☐ 86580	TB Intradermal Test	
☐ 86585	TB Tine Test	
☐ 87070	Culture	
☐ 70190	X-Ray; Optic Foramina	
☐ 70210	X-Ray Sinuses Complete	
☐ 71010	Radiological Exam Ent Spine	
☐ 71020	X-Ray Chest Pa & Lat	
☐ 72050	X-Ray Spine, Cerv (4 views)	
☐ 72090	X-Ray Spine; Scoliosis Ex	
☐ 72110	Spine, lumbosacral; a/p & Lat	
☐ 73030	Shoulder-Comp, min w/ 2vws	
☐ 73070	Elbow, anteropost & later vws	
☐ 73120	X-Ray; Hand, 2 views	
☐ 73560	X-Ray, Knee, 1 or 2 views	
☐ 74022	X-Ray; Abdomen, Complete	
☐ 75552	Cardiac Magnetic Res Img	
☐ 76020	X-Ray; Bone Age Studies	
☐ 77054	Mammary Ductogram Complete	
☐ 78465	Myocardial Perfusion Img	

☐ CPT	DESCRIPTION	FEE
PROCEDURES/TESTS		
☐ 00452	Anesthesia for Rad Surgery	
☐ 11100	Skin Biopsy	
☐ 15852	Dressing Change	
☐ 29075	Cast Appl. - Lower Arm	
☐ 29530	Strapping of Knee	
☐ 29705	Removal/Revis of Cast w/Exa	
☐ 53670	Catheterization Incl. Suppl	
☐ 57452	Colposcopy	
☐ 57505	ECC	
☐ 69420	Myringotomy	
☐ 92081	Visual Field Examination	
☐ 92100	Serial Tonometry Exam	
☐ 92120	Tonography	
☐ 92552	Pure Tone Audiometry	
☐ 92567	Tympanometry	
☐ 93000	Electrocardiogram	
☐ 93015	Exercise Stress Test (ETT)	
☐ 93017	ETT Tracing Only	
☐ 93040	Electrocardiogram - Rhythm	
☐ 96100	Psychological Testing	
☐ 99000	Specimen Handling	
☐ 99058	Office Emergency Care	
☐ 99070	Surgical Tray - Misc.	
☐ 99080	Special Reports of Med Rec	
☐ 99195	Phlebotomy	
☐	_____	
☐	_____	
☐	_____	

☐	ICD-9 CODE DIAGNOSIS	
☐ 009.0	Infect. colitis, enteritis, & gastroenteritis	
☐ 133.0	Scabies	
☐ 174.9	Breast Cancer, Female, Unspecified	
☐ 185	Malignant neoplasm of prostate	
☐ 250.00	Diabetes Mellitus w/o mention of Complication	
☐ 272.4	Hyperlipidemia	
☐ 282.5	Anemia, Sickle-cell Trait	
☐ 282.60	Sickle-cell disease, unspecified	
☐ 285.9	Anemia, Unspecified	
☐ 300.4	Dysthymic disorder	
☐ 340	Multiple Sclerosis	
☐ 342.90	Hemiplegia - Unspec.	
☐ 346.90	Migraine, unspecified	
☐ 352.9	Unspecified disorder of cranial nerves	
☐ 354.0	Carpal Tunnel Syndrome	
☐ 355.0	Sciatic Nerve Root Lesion	
☐ 366.9	Cataract	
☒ 386.00	Menier's disease, unspecified	
☐ 401.1	Essential Hypertension, Benign	
☐ 414.9	Ischemic Heart Disease	
☐ 428.0	Congestive Heart Failure (CHF), unspecified	

☐	ICD-9 CODE DIAGNOSIS	
☐ 435.0	Basilar Artery Syndrome	
☐ 440.0	Atherosclerosis	
☐ 442.81	Carotid Artery	
☐ 460	Common Cold (Acute Nasopharyngitis)	
☐ 461.9	Acute Sinusitis	
☐ 474.00	Chronic Tonsillitis & Adenoiditis	
☐ 477.9	Allergic Rhinitis, Cause Unspecified	
☐ 487.0	Influenza with pneumonia	
☐ 496	Chronic Airway Obstruction	
☐ 522.0	Pulpitis	
☐ 524.60	Temporo-Mandibular Joint Disorder - Unspec.	
☐ 536.8	Stomach Pain	
☐ 553.3	Hiatal Hernia	
☐ 564.1	Spastic Colon	
☐ 574.40	Chronic Hepatitis, Unspecified	
☐ 571.5	Cirrhosis of Liver w/o mention of alcohol	
☐ 573.3	Hepatitis	
☐ 575.2	Obstruction of Gallbladder	
☐ 648.20	Anemia - Compl. Pregnancy	
☐ 715.90	Osteoarthritis - Unspec.	
☐ 721.3	Lumbar Osteo/Spondylarthrit	

☐	ICD-9 CODE DIAGNOSIS	
☐ 724.2	Pain: Lower Back	
☐ 727.67	Rupture of Achilles Tendon	
☐ 780.1	Hallucinations	
☐ 780.3	Convulsions, Other	
☐ 780.50	Sleep Disturbances, Unspecified	
☐ 783.0	Anorexia	
☐ 783.1	Abnormal Weight Gain	
☐ 783.21	Abnormal Weight Loss	
☐ 823.80	Fractured Tibia	
☐ 823.81	Fractured Fibula	
☐ 831.00	Dislocated Shoulder, Closed, Unspecified	
☐ 835.00	Dislocated Hip, Closed, Unspecified	
☐ 842.00	Sprained Wrist, Unspecified Site	
☐ 845.00	Sprained Ankle, Unspecified Site	
☐ 919.5	Insect Bite, Nonvenomous	
☐ 921.1	Contus Eyelid/Perioc Area	
☐ v16.3	Fam. Hist of Breast Cancer	
☐ v17.4	Fam. Hist of Cardiovasc Dis	
☐ v20.2	Well Child	
☐ v22.0	Pregnancy - First Normal	
☐ v22.1	Pregnancy - Normal	

Previous Balance	Today's Charges	Total Due	Amount Paid	New Balance
_____			$10 check #1029	

Follow Up

PRN _____ Weeks _____ Months _____ Units _____

Next Appointment Date: _____   Time: _____

I hereby authorize release of any information acquired in the course of
examination or treatment and allow a photocopy of my signature to be used.

_____

Figure 6-6 Two Procedures Posted – Ramirez

```
M Student: Lois Fitzpatrick                                                    _ □ ✕
File  Edit  View  Windows  Help

  Patient #: 320.0     [Leanna Ramirez              ]     Dept.   :  0
  Voucher #: 1344             Doctor #  :  1 Monroe MD, James   Location :
                              Supervisor:  1 Monroe MD, James

  Dates    P.O.S.  Procedure   Modifier Diag. 1-4    Units      Charges    T.O.S.

  06/02/08  3        ■ . . . . . . . . . .                . . . . .  $    15.00  1

  |Blood Count, Manual Cell Count       | 386.00    Menier's disease, unspecified |
  Comment:                              | . . . . . . . . .                        |
                                        | . . . . . . . . .                        |
  Ins: Primary#: 7.0        Assign: Y    Secondary#: 0.0       EMC Billable: Y
  [Posted]
        Date      Co #  Dr# Procedure  Diag       Units      Charges   Total Chgs

    1  06/02/08 7    1   99213      386.00      1.00       40.00      40.00
    2  06/02/08 7    1   85032      386.00      1.00       15.00      55.00




     Enter '?', '!', '?code' for Help, '?~' for Macros, or '%' for Standing Orders

Ready                                                              NUM     ↑↓⇔⇒
```

Figure 6-7 Check from Patient – Ramirez

```
┌──────────────────────────────────────────────────────────────────────────────┐
│                                                                                │
│  Michael and Leanna Ramirez                                        1029        │
│  25-12 Blossom Street                                                          │
│  Sacramento, CA 94056                    June 2            20 08               │
│                                        ─────────────────                       │
│                                                                                │
│  Pay to the                                                                    │
│  order of  ____Sydney Carrington & Associates_____  $ | 10.00 |              │
│                                                                                │
│              ____Ten and 00/100_____      Dollars           │
│                                                                                │
│  FIRST COMMUNITY BANK                                                          │
│  Madison, California                                                           │
│                                                                                │
│  Memo  _____        Leanna Ramirez                           │
│  ⑆153154403⑆  45385⑈  1029                                                     │
│                                                                                │
└──────────────────────────────────────────────────────────────────────────────┘
```

Figure 6-8 Patient Visit Copay

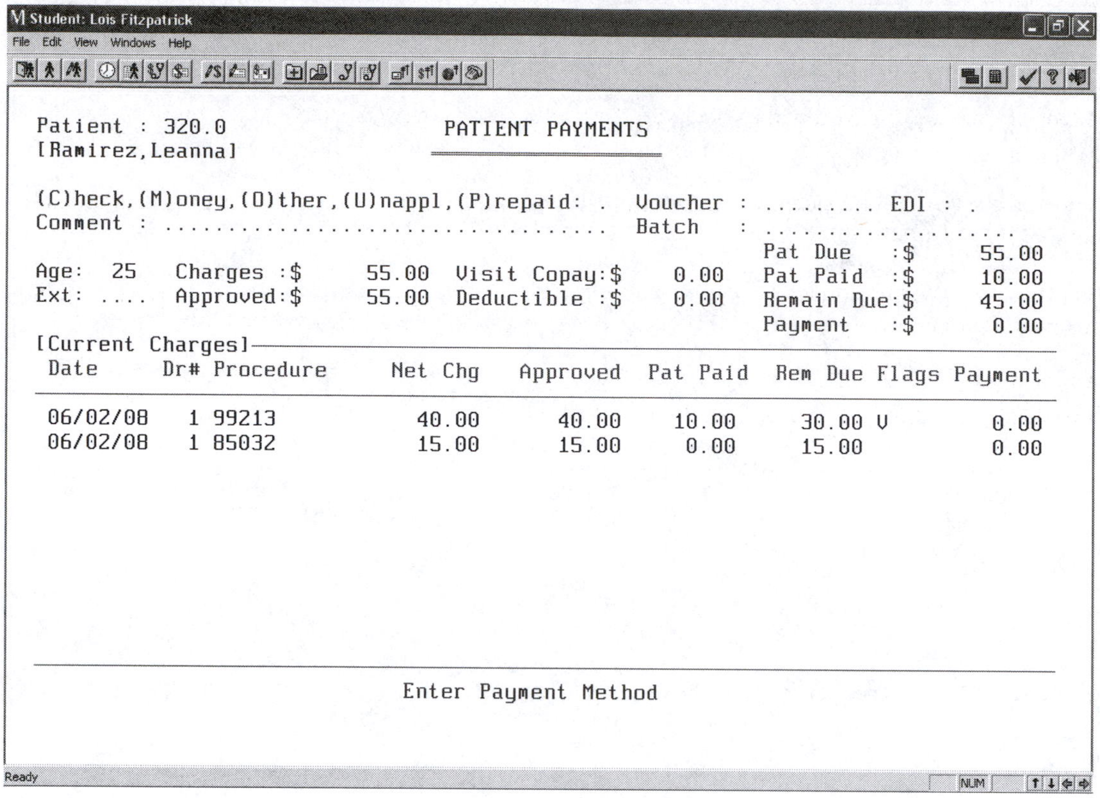

```
M Student: Lois Fitzpatrick                                          _ ☐ ✕
File  Edit  View  Windows  Help
[toolbar icons]                                              ▣ ▣ ✓ ? ◄

  Patient : 320.0              PATIENT PAYMENTS
  [Ramirez,Leanna]

  (C)heck,(M)oney,(O)ther,(U)nappl,(P)repaid: .   Voucher : ........ EDI : .
  Comment : ...............................    Batch  : ................
                                                          Pat Due   :$    55.00
  Age:  25    Charges :$   55.00  Visit Copay:$   0.00   Pat Paid  :$    10.00
  Ext:  ....  Approved:$   55.00  Deductible :$   0.00   Remain Due:$    45.00
                                                          Payment   :$     0.00
  [Current Charges]─────────────────────────────────────
  Date      Dr# Procedure    Net Chg   Approved  Pat Paid  Rem Due Flags Payment

  06/02/08   1 99213          40.00     40.00     10.00     30.00 V      0.00
  06/02/08   1 85032          15.00     15.00      0.00     15.00        0.00




  ─────────────────────────────────────────────────────────
                    Enter Payment Method

Ready                                                     NUM    ↑↓↔
```

EXERCISE 3: PAYMENT ENTRY

ANNA MARCHESE; ACCOUNT 321

GOAL(S): In this exercise, you will post a procedure and post a payment from the Payment Entry screen for Anna Marchese, who will pay in full for her visit.

1. Before posting your entry, study the encounter form in Figure 6-9. Note the charge and diagnosis before attempting the data entry.

2. Based on the information found on the encounter form, post the charge for Anna Marchese. Compare your screen to Figure 6-10, then <Process> the screen and exit the Procedure Entry screen.

3. Anna Marchese comes back later that day to give you a check for her visit. See Figure 6-11. Apply the $40 check to her account. Compare your screen to Figure 6-12 before you press the F1 key.

Figure 6-9 Encounter Form – Marchese

Sydney Carrington & Associates P.A.
34 Sycamore Street Suite 300
Madison, CA 95653

Date: 06/02/2008

Voucher No.: 1011

Time:

Patient: Anna Marchese
Guarantor:

Patient No: 321.0
Doctor: 3 – S. Carrington

□ CPT	DESCRIPTION	FEE
OFFICE/HOSPITAL CONSULTS		
□ 99201	Office New:Focused Hx-Exam	
□ 99202	Office New:Expanded Hx.Exam	
□ 99211	Office Estb:Min./None Hx-Exa	
□ 99212	Office Estb:Focused Hx-Exam	
☒ 99213	Office Estb:Expanded Hx-Exa	$40
□ 99214	Office Estb:Detailed Hx-Exa	
□ 99215	Office Estb:Comprhn Hx-Exam	
□ 99221	Hosp. Initial:Comprh Hx-	
□ 99223	Hosp. Ini:Comprh Hx-Exam/Hi	
□ 99231	Hosp. Subsequent: S-Fwd	
□ 99232	Hosp. Subsequent: Comprhn Hx	
□ 99233	Hosp. Subsequent: Ex/Hi	
□ 99238	Hospital Visit Discharge Ex	
□ 99371	Telephone Consult - Simple	
□ 99372	Telephone Consult - Intermed	
□ 99373	Telephone Consult - Complex	
□ 90840	Counseling - 25 minutes	
□ 90806	Counseling - 50 minutes	
□ 90865	Counseling - Special Interview	
IMMUNIZATIONS/INJECTIONS		
□ 90585	BCG Vaccine	
□ 90659	Influenza Virus Vaccine	
□ 90701	Immunization-DTP	
□ 90702	DT Vaccine	
□ 90703	Tetanus Toxoids	
□ 90732	Pneumococcal Vaccine	
□ 90746	Hepatitis B Vaccine	
□ 90749	Immunization: Unlisted	

□ CPT	DESCRIPTION	FEE
LABORATORY/RADIOLOGY		
□ 81000	Urinalysis	
□ 81002	Urinalysis; Pregnancy Test	
□ 82951	Glucose Tolerance Test	
□ 84478	Triglycerides	
□ 84550	Uric Acid: Blood Chemistry	
□ 84830	Ovulation Test	
□ 85014	Hematocrit	
□ 85032	Hemogram, Complete Blood Wk	
□ 86403	Particle Agglutination Test	
□ 86485	Skin Test; Candida	
□ 86580	TB Intradermal Test	
□ 86585	TB Tine Test	
□ 87070	Culture	
□ 70190	X-Ray; Optic Foramina	
□ 70210	X-Ray Sinuses Complete	
□ 71010	Radiological Exam Ent Spine	
□ 71020	X-Ray Chest Pa & Lat	
□ 72050	X-Ray Spine, Cerv (4 views)	
□ 72090	X-Ray Spine; Scoliosis Ex	
□ 72110	Spine, lumbosacral; a/p & Lat	
□ 73030	Shoulder-Comp, min w/ 2vws	
□ 73070	Elbow, anteropost & later vws	
□ 73120	X-Ray; Hand, 2 views	
□ 73560	X-Ray, Knee, 1 or 2 views	
□ 74022	X-Ray; Abdomen, Complete	
□ 75552	Cardiac Magnetic Res Img	
□ 76020	X-Ray; Bone Age Studies	
□ 77054	Mammary Ductogram Complete	
□ 78465	Myocardial Perfusion Img	

□ CPT	DESCRIPTION	FEE
PROCEDURES/TESTS		
□ 00452	Anesthesia for Rad Surgery	
□ 11100	Skin Biopsy	
□ 15852	Dressing Change	
□ 29075	Cast Appl. - Lower Arm	
□ 29530	Strapping of Knee	
□ 29705	Removal/Revis of Cast w/Exa	
□ 53670	Catheterization Incl. Suppl	
□ 57452	Colposcopy	
□ 57505	ECC	
□ 69420	Myringotomy	
□ 92081	Visual Field Examination	
□ 92100	Serial Tonometry Exam	
□ 92120	Tonography	
□ 92552	Pure Tone Audiometry	
□ 92567	Tympanometry	
□ 93000	Electrocardiogram	
□ 93015	Exercise Stress Test (ETT)	
□ 93017	ETT Tracing Only	
□ 93040	Electrocardiogram - Rhythm	
□ 96100	Psychological Testing	
□ 99000	Specimen Handling	
□ 99058	Office Emergency Care	
□ 99070	Surgical Tray - Misc.	
□ 99080	Special Reports of Med Rec	
□ 99195	Phlebotomy	
□ _____	_____	
□ _____	_____	
□ _____	_____	
□ _____	_____	

□	ICD-9 CODE DIAGNOSIS
□ 009.0	Infect. colitis, enteritis, & gastroenteritis
□ 133.0	Scabies
□ 174.9	Breast Cancer, Female, Unspecified
□ 185	Malignant neoplasm of prostate
□ 250.00	Diabetes Mellitus w/o mention of Complication
□ 272.4	Hyperlipidemia
□ 282.5	Anemia, Sickle-cell Trait
□ 282.60	Sickle-cell disease, unspecified
□ 285.9	Anemia, Unspecified
□ 300.4	Dysthymic disorder
□ 340	Multiple Sclerosis
□ 342.90	Hemiplegia - Unspec.
□ 346.90	Migraine, unspecified
□ 352.9	Unspecified disorder of cranial nerves
□ 354.0	Carpal Tunnel Syndrome
□ 355.0	Sciatic Nerve Root Lesion
□ 366.9	Cataract
□ 386.00	Menier's disease, unspecified
□ 401.1	Essential Hypertension, Benign
□ 414.9	Ischemic Heart Disease
□ 428.0	Congestive Heart Failure (CHF), unspecified

□	ICD-9 CODE DIAGNOSIS
□ 435.0	Basilar Artery Syndrome
□ 440.0	Atherosclerosis
□ 442.81	Carotid Artery
□ 460	Common Cold (Acute Nasopharyngitis)
☒ 461.9	Acute Sinusitis
□ 474.00	Chronic Tonsillitis & Adenoiditis
□ 477.9	Allergic Rhinitis, Cause Unspecified
□ 487.0	Influenza with pneumonia
□ 496	Chronic Airway Obstruction
□ 522.0	Pulpitis
□ 524.60	Temporo-Mandibular Joint Disorder - Unspec.
□ 536.8	Stomach Pain
□ 553.3	Hiatal Hernia
□ 564.1	Spastic Colon
□ 574.40	Chronic Hepatitis, Unspecified
□ 571.5	Cirrhosis of Liver w/o mention of alcohol
□ 573.3	Hepatitis
□ 575.2	Obstruction of Gallbladder
□ 648.20	Anemia - Compl. Pregnancy
□ 715.90	Osteoarthritis - Unspec.
□ 721.3	Lumbar Osteo/Spondylarthrit

□	ICD-9 CODE DIAGNOSIS
□ 724.2	Pain: Lower Back
□ 727.67	Rupture of Achilles Tendon
□ 780.1	Hallucinations
□ 780.3	Convulsions, Other
□ 780.50	Sleep Disturbances, Unspecified
□ 783.0	Anorexia
□ 783.1	Abnormal Weight Gain
□ 783.21	Abnormal Weight Loss
□ 823.80	Fractured Tibia
□ 823.81	Fractured Fibula
□ 831.00	Dislocated Shoulder, Closed, Unspecified
□ 835.00	Dislocated Hip, Closed, Unspecified
□ 842.00	Sprained Wrist, Unspecified Site
□ 845.00	Sprained Ankle, Unspecified Site
□ 919.5	Insect Bite, Nonvenomous
□ 921.1	Contus Eyelid/Perioc Area
□ v16.3	Fam. Hist of Breast Cancer
□ v17.4	Fam. Hist of Cardiovasc Dis
□ v20.2	Well Child
□ v22.0	Pregnancy - First Normal
□ v22.1	Pregnancy - Normal

Previous Balance	Today's Charges	Total Due	Amount Paid	New Balance
_____	_____	_____	$40 check #103	

Follow Up

PRN _____ Weeks _____   Months _____ Units _____

Next Appointment Date: _____   Time: _____

I hereby authorize release of any information acquired in the course of
examination or treatment and allow a photocopy of my signature to be used.

_____   _____

_____   _____

Figure 6-10 Procedure Entry – No Insurance

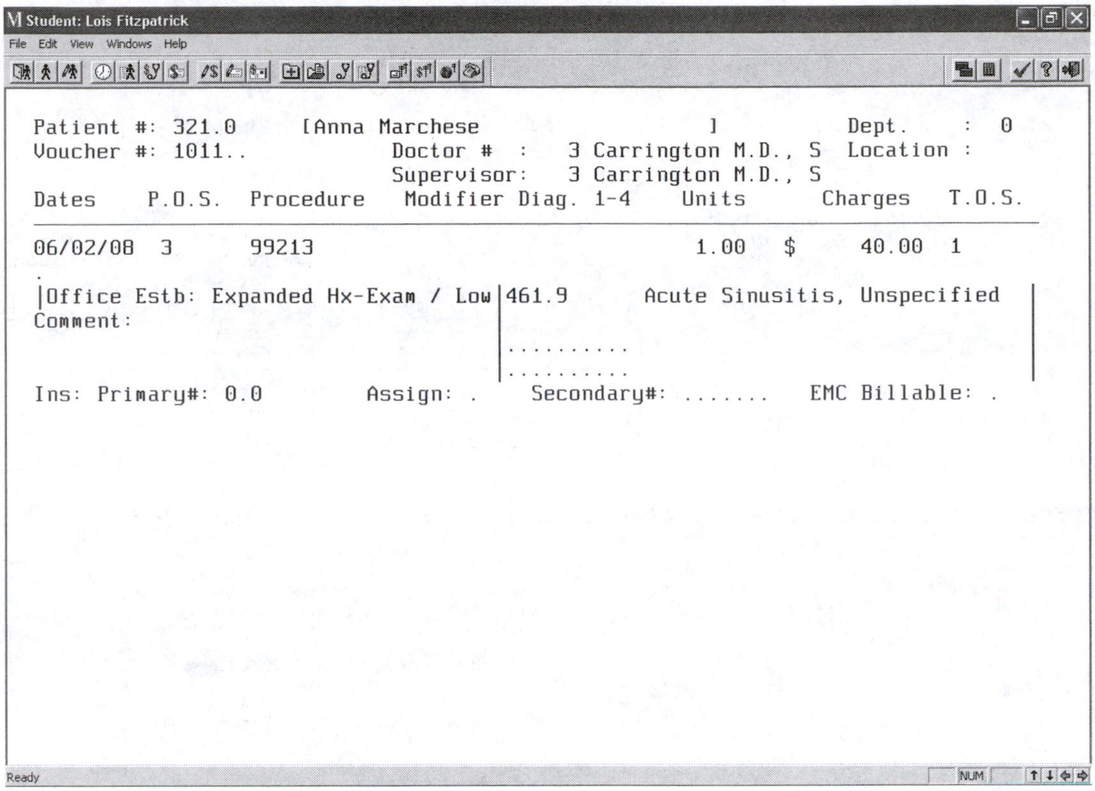

```
M Student: Lois Fitzpatrick                                              _ |F|X
File  Edit  View  Windows  Help

Patient #: 321.0      [Anna Marchese              ]       Dept.   :  0
Voucher #: 1011..              Doctor # :  3 Carrington M.D., S Location :
                               Supervisor:  3 Carrington M.D., S
Dates    P.O.S.  Procedure   Modifier Diag. 1-4   Units      Charges   T.O.S.
──────────────────────────────────────────────────────────────────────
06/02/08  3      99213                          1.00  $    40.00  1
.
|Office Estb: Expanded Hx-Exam / Low|461.9     Acute Sinusitis, Unspecified |
Comment:
                                   |..........
                                   |..........
Ins: Primary#: 0.0        Assign: .   Secondary#: .......  EMC Billable: .




Ready                                                    NUM      ↑↓⇦⇨
```

Figure 6-11 Check from Patient – Marchese

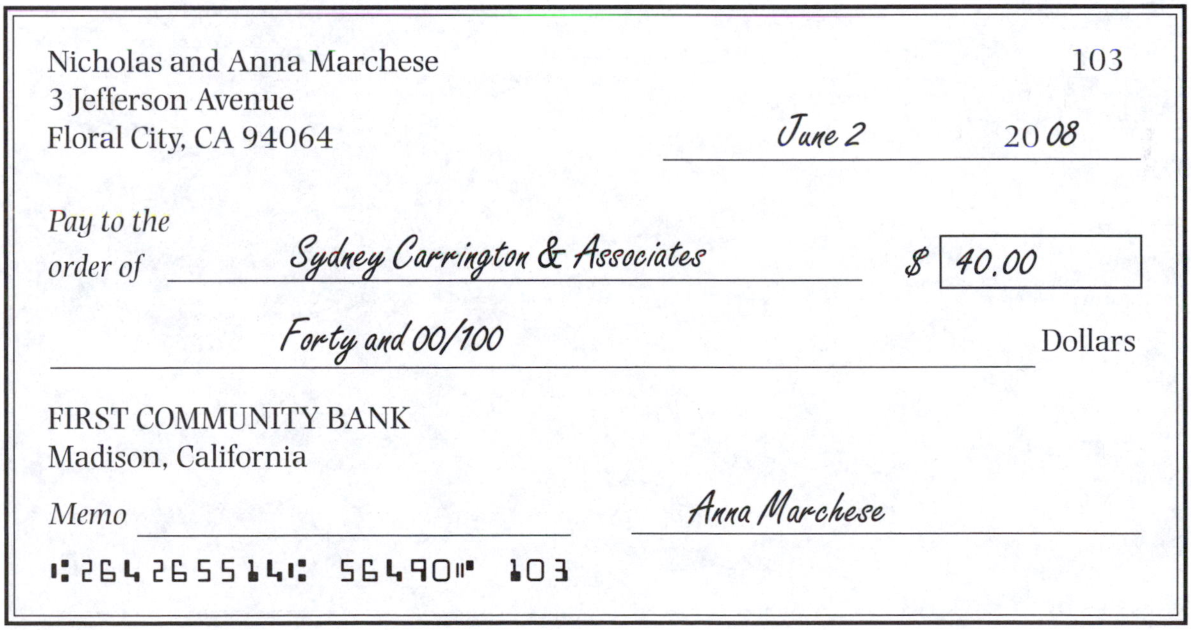

```
┌─────────────────────────────────────────────────────────────────┐
│ Nicholas and Anna Marchese                              103       │
│ 3 Jefferson Avenue                                                │
│ Floral City, CA 94064              June 2        20 08            │
│                                  _____  _____  │
│ Pay to the                                                        │
│ order of    Sydney Carrington & Associates      $ │ 40.00 │       │
│ _____              │
│             Forty and 00/100                         Dollars      │
│ _____               │
│ FIRST COMMUNITY BANK                                              │
│ Madison, California                                               │
│ Memo _____    Anna Marchese _____     │
│ ⑆264265514⑆ 56490⑈ 103                                           │
└─────────────────────────────────────────────────────────────────┘
```

Figure 6-12 Payment Entry Before Posting

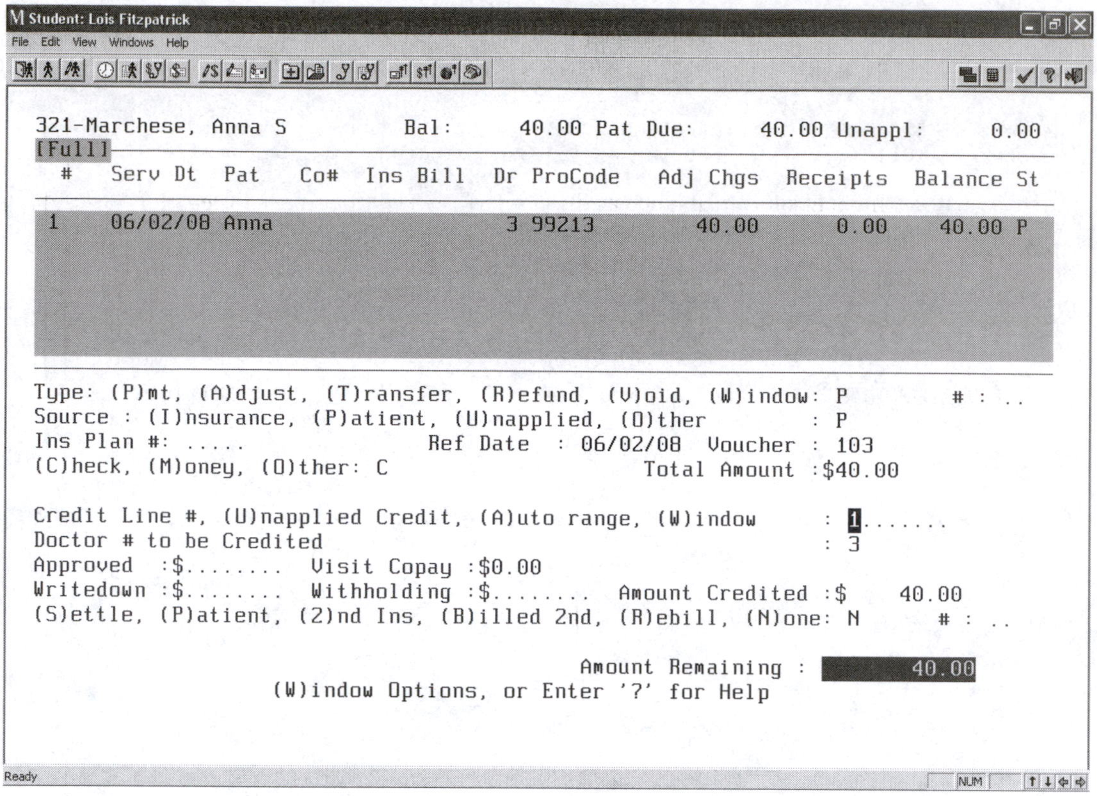

EXERCISE 4: APPLYING COPAYMENTS

PAUL SANTOS; CAROL SANTOS; ACCOUNT 322

GOAL(S): In this exercise, you will post procedures and post a payment from the Payment Entry screen for Paul and Carol Santos who will pay their copayments.

Paul and Carol Santos have Epsilon insurance and must pay an $8 copayment for each visit. Paul Santos was seen by the doctor early in the day. He left without paying his $8 copayment. Later that same day, Carol Santos was also seen by the doctor. After her visit, she gives a check in the amount of $16 for both copayments.

1. Before posting your entry, study the encounter form in Figure 6-13. Note the charges and before attempting the data entry.

2. Based on the information found on the encounter form, post the charges for Paul Santos. Compare your screen to Figure 6-14, then EXIT the Procedure Entry screen.

Figure 6-13   Encounter Form – Paul Santos

Sydney Carrington & Associates P.A.
34 Sycamore Street Suite 300
Madison, CA 95653

Date: 06/02/2008   Voucher No.: 906

Time:

Patient: Paul Santos   Patient No: 322.0
Guarantor: Doctor: 2 – F. Simpson

	CPT	DESCRIPTION	FEE		CPT	DESCRIPTION	FEE		CPT	DESCRIPTION	FEE
OFFICE/HOSPITAL CONSULTS				**LABORATORY/RADIOLOGY**				**PROCEDURES/TESTS**			
☐	99201	Office New:Focused Hx-Exam		☐	81000	Urinalysis		☐	00452	Anesthesia for Rad Surgery	
☐	99202	Office New:Expanded Hx.Exam		☐	81002	Urinalysis; Pregnancy Test		☐	11100	Skin Biopsy	
☐	99211	Offlce Estb:Min./None Hx-Exa		☐	82951	Glucose Tolerance Test		☐	15852	Dressing Change	
☐	99212	Office Estb:Focused Hx-Exam		☐	84478	Triglycerides		☐	29075	Cast Appl. - Lower Arm	
☒	99213	Office Estb:Expanded Hx-Exa	$40	☐	84550	Uric Acid: Blood Chemistry		☐	29530	Strapping of Knee	
☐	99214	Office Estb:Detailed Hx-Exa		☐	84830	Ovulation Test		☐	29705	Removal/Revis of Cast w/Exa	
☐	99215	Office Estb:Comprhn Hx-Exam		☐	85014	Hematocrit		☐	53670	Catheterization Incl. Suppl	
☐	99221	Hosp. Initial:Comprh Hx-		☐	85032	Hemogram, Complete Blood Wk		☐	57452	Colposcopy	
☐	99223	Hosp. Ini:Comprh Hx-Exam/Hi		☐	86403	Particle Agglutination Test		☐	57505	ECC	
☐	99231	Hosp. Subsequent: S-Fwd		☐	86485	Skin Test; Candida		☐	69420	Myringotomy	
☐	99232	Hosp. Subsequent: Comprhn Hx		☐	86580	TB Intradermal Test		☐	92081	Visual Field Examination	
☐	99233	Hosp. Subsequent: Ex/Hi		☐	86585	TB Tine Test		☐	92100	Serial Tonometry Exam	
☐	99238	Hospital Visit Discharge Ex		☐	87070	Culture		☐	92120	Tonography	
☐	99371	Telephone Consult - Simple		☐	70190	X-Ray; Optic Foramina		☐	92552	Pure Tone Audiometry	
☐	99372	Telephone Consult - Intermed		☐	70210	X-Ray Sinuses Complete		☐	92567	Tympanometry	
☐	99373	Telephone Consult - Complex		☐	71010	Radiological Exam Ent Spine		☒	93000	Electrocardiogram	$57
☐	90840	Counseling - 25 minutes		☐	71020	X-Ray Chest Pa & Lat		☐	93015	Exercise Stress Test (ETT)	
☐	90806	Counseling - 50 minutes		☐	72050	X-Ray Spine, Cerv (4 views)		☐	93017	ETT Tracing Only	
☐	90865	Counseling - Special Interview		☐	72090	X-Ray Spine; Scoliosis Ex		☐	93040	Electrocardiogram - Rhythm	
				☐	72110	Spine, lumbosacral; a/p & Lat		☐	96100	Psychological Testing	
IMMUNIZATIONS/INJECTIONS				☐	73030	Shoulder-Comp, min w/ 2vws		☐	99000	Specimen Handling	
☐	90585	BCG Vaccine		☐	73070	Elbow, anteropost & later vws		☐	99058	Office Emergency Care	
☐	90659	Influenza Virus Vaccine		☐	73120	X-Ray; Hand, 2 views		☐	99070	Surgical Tray - Misc.	
☐	90701	Immunization-DTP		☐	73560	X-Ray, Knee, 1 or 2 views		☐	99080	Special Reports of Med Rec	
☐	90702	DT Vaccine		☐	74022	X-Ray; Abdomen, Complete		☐	99195	Phlebotomy	
☐	90703	Tetanus Toxoids		☐	75552	Cardiac Magnetic Res Img		☐		_____	
☐	90732	Pneumococcal Vaccine		☐	76020	X-Ray; Bone Age Studies		☐		_____	
☐	90746	Hepatitis B Vaccine		☐	77054	Mammary Ductogram Complete		☐		_____	
☐	90749	Immunization: Unlisted		☐	78465	Myocardial Perfusion Img		☐		_____	

	ICD-9 CODE DIAGNOSIS			ICD-9 CODE DIAGNOSIS			ICD-9 CODE DIAGNOSIS	
☐	009.0	Infect. colitis, enteritis, & gastroenteritis	☐	435.0	Basilar Artery Syndrome	☐	724.2	Pain: Lower Back
☐	133.0	Scabies	☐	440.0	Atherosclerosis	☐	727.67	Rupture of Achilles Tendon
☐	174.9	Breast Cancer, Female, Unspecified	☐	442.81	Carotid Artery	☐	780.1	Hallucinations
☐	185	Malignant neoplasm of prostate	☐	460	Common Cold (Acute Nasopharyngitis)	☐	780.3	Convulsions, Other
☐	250.00	Diabetes Mellitus w/o mention of Complication	☐	461.9	Acute Sinusitis	☐	780.50	Sleep Disturbances, Unspecified
☐	272.4	Hyperlipidemia	☐	474.00	Chronic Tonsillitis & Adenoiditis	☐	783.0	Anorexia
☐	282.5	Anemia, Sickle-cell Trait	☐	477.9	Allergic Rhinitis, Cause Unspecified	☐	783.1	Abnormal Weight Gain
☐	282.60	Sickle-cell disease, unspecified	☐	487.0	Influenza with pneumonia	☐	783.21	Abnormal Weight Loss
☐	285.9	Anemia, Unspecified	☐	496	Chronic Airway Obstruction	☐	823.80	Fractured Tibia
☐	300.4	Dysthymic disorder	☐	522.0	Pulpitis	☐	823.81	Fractured Fibula
☐	340	Multiple Sclerosis	☐	524.60	Temporo-Mandibular Joint Disorder - Unspec.	☐	831.00	Dislocated Shoulder, Closed, Unspecified
☐	342.90	Hemiplegia - Unspec.	☐	536.8	Stomach Pain	☐	835.00	Dislocated Hip, Closed, Unspecified
☐	346.90	Migraine, unspecified	☐	553.3	Hiatal Hernia	☐	842.00	Sprained Wrist, Unspecified Site
☐	352.9	Unspecified disorder of cranial nerves	☐	564.1	Spastic Colon	☐	845.00	Sprained Ankle, Unspecified Site
☐	354.0	Carpal Tunnel Syndrome	☐	574.40	Chronic Hepatitis, Unspecified	☐	919.5	Insect Bite, Nonvenomous
☐	355.0	Sclatic Nerve Root Lesion	☐	571.5	Cirrhosis of Liver w/o mention of alcohol	☐	921.1	Contus Eyelid/Perioc Area
☐	366.9	Cataract	☐	573.3	Hepatitis	☐	v16.3	Fam. Hist of Breast Cancer
☐	386.00	Menier's disease, unspecified	☐	575.2	Obstruction of Gallbladder	☐	v17.4	Fam. Hist of Cardiovasc Dis
☐	401.1	Essential Hypertension, Benign	☐	648.20	Anemia - Compl. Pregnancy	☐	v20.2	Well Child
☐	414.9	Ischemic Heart Disease	☐	715.90	Osteoarthritis - Unspec.	☐	v22.0	Pregnancy - First Normal
☐	428.0	Congestive Heart Failure (CHF), unspecified	☐	721.3	Lumbar Osteo/Spondylarthrit	☐	v22.1	Pregnancy - Normal
						X	786.50	Chest Pain

Previous Balance	Today's Charges	Total Due	Amount Paid	New Balance
_____	_____	_____	_____	_____

Follow Up

PRN _____ Weeks _____ Months _____ Units _____

Next Appointment Date: Time:

I hereby authorize release of any information acquired in the course of
examination or treatment and allow a photocopy of my signature to be used.

_____   _____

Figure 6-14   Posted Procedures – Santos

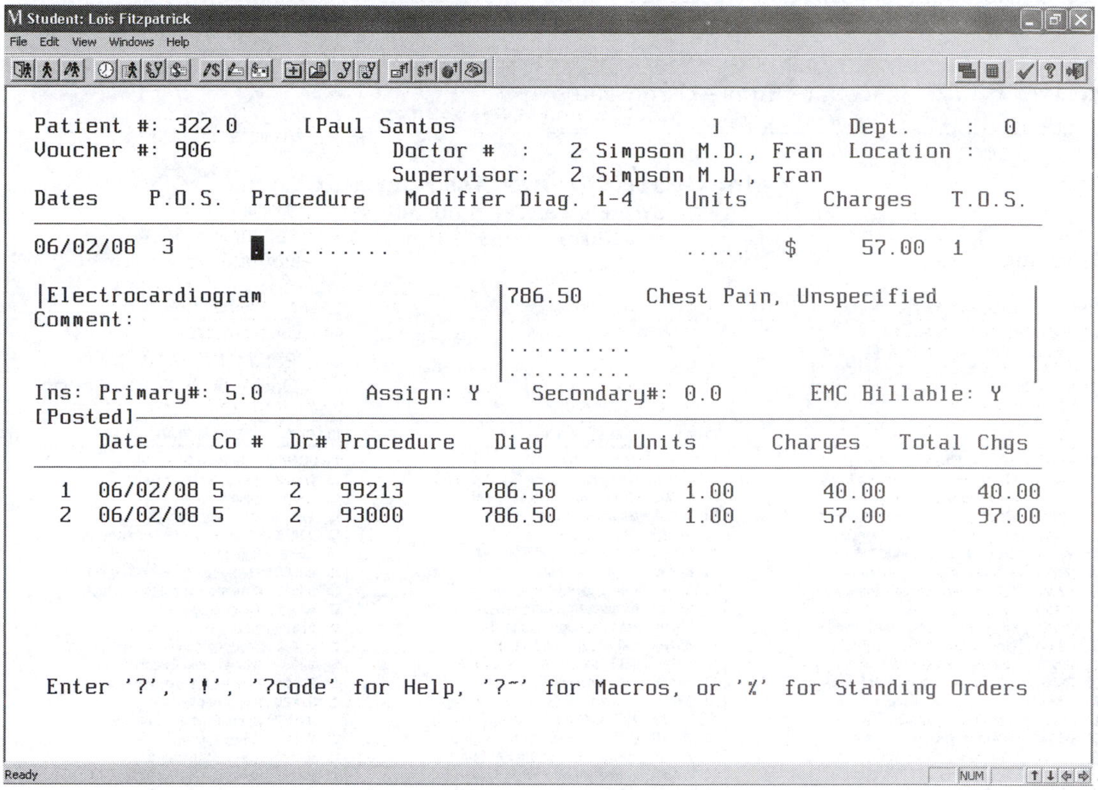

```
M Student: Lois Fitzpatrick                                              _ ⊡ ✕
File  Edit  View  Windows  Help

 ☐🕮 🕮🕮  ⊙🕮🕮🕮  🕮🕮🕮  🕮🕮🕮🕮  🕮🕮🕮🕮                            🕮🕮  ✓ ? 🕮

   Patient #: 322.0     [Paul Santos                   ]      Dept.    :  0
   Voucher #: 906                 Doctor #  :   2 Simpson M.D., Fran  Location :
                                  Supervisor:   2 Simpson M.D., Fran
   Dates     P.O.S.   Procedure   Modifier Diag. 1-4    Units       Charges   T.O.S.
  _____
   06/02/08  3      █..........                      ..... $     57.00  1

   |Electrocardiogram                    |786.50     Chest Pain, Unspecified   |
   Comment:                              |
                                         |..........
                                         |..........
   Ins: Primary#: 5.0        Assign: Y     Secondary#: 0.0      EMC Billable: Y
   [Posted]————————————————————————————————————————————————————————————————
        Date     Co #  Dr# Procedure   Diag      Units     Charges   Total Chgs
  _____
     1  06/02/08 5     2   99213       786.50     1.00      40.00     40.00
     2  06/02/08 5     2   93000       786.50     1.00      57.00     97.00




   Enter '?', '!', '?code' for Help, '?~' for Macros, or '%' for Standing Orders


 Ready                                                          NUM    ↑↓⇦⇨
```

3. Select Carol Santos and based on the information on her encounter form (Figure 6-15), post one charge for her. Compare your screen to Figure 6-16, then EXIT Procedure Entry.

Figure 6-15 Encounter Form – Carol Santos

Sydney Carrington & Associates P.A.
34 Sycamore Street Suite 300
Madison, CA 95653

Date: 06/02/2008   Voucher No.: 1215

Time:

Patient: Carol Santos   Patient No: 322.1
Guarantor: Doctor: 2 – F. Simpson

□ CPT	DESCRIPTION	FEE	□ CPT	DESCRIPTION	FEE	□ CPT	DESCRIPTION	FEE
OFFICE/HOSPITAL CONSULTS			**LABORATORY/RADIOLOGY**			**PROCEDURES/TESTS**		
□ 99201	Office New:Focused Hx-Exam		□ 81000	Urinalysis		□ 00452	Anesthesia for Rad Surgery	
□ 99202	Office New:Expanded Hx.Exam		□ 81002	Urinalysis; Pregnancy Test		□ 11100	Skin Biopsy	
□ 99211	Office Estb:Min./None Hx-Exa		□ 82951	Glucose Tolerance Test		□ 15852	Dressing Change	
□ 99212	Office Estb:Focused Hx-Exam		□ 84478	Triglycerides		□ 29075	Cast Appl. - Lower Arm	
□ 99213	Office Estb:Expanded Hx-Exa		□ 84550	Uric Acid: Blood Chemistry		□ 29530	Strapping of Knee	
☒ 99214	Office Estb:Detailed Hx-Exa	$50	□ 84830	Ovulation Test		□ 29705	Removal/Revis of Cast w/Exa	
□ 99215	Office Estb:Comprhn Hx-Exam		□ 85014	Hematocrit		□ 53670	Catheterization Incl. Suppl	
□ 99221	Hosp. Initial:Comprh Hx-		□ 85032	Hemogram, Complete Blood Wk		□ 57452	Colposcopy	
□ 99223	Hosp. Ini:Comprh Hx-Exam/Hi		□ 86403	Particle Agglutination Test		□ 57505	ECC	
□ 99231	Hosp. Subsequent: S-Fwd		□ 86485	Skin Test; Candida		□ 69420	Myringotomy	
□ 99232	Hosp. Subsequent: Comprhn Hx		□ 86580	TB Intradermal Test		□ 92081	Visual Field Examination	
□ 99233	Hosp. Subsequent: Ex/Hi		□ 86585	TB Tine Test		□ 92100	Serial Tonometry Exam	
□ 99238	Hospital Visit Discharge Ex		□ 87070	Culture		□ 92120	Tonography	
□ 99371	Telephone Consult - Simple		□ 70190	X-Ray; Optic Foramina		□ 92552	Pure Tone Audiometry	
□ 99372	Telephone Consult - Intermed		□ 70210	X-Ray Sinuses Complete		□ 92567	Tympanometry	
□ 99373	Telephone Consult - Complex		□ 71010	Radiological Exam Ent Spine		□ 93000	Electrocardiogram	
□ 90840	Counseling - 25 minutes		□ 71020	X-Ray Chest Pa & Lat		□ 93015	Exercise Stress Test (ETT)	
□ 90806	Counseling - 50 minutes		□ 72050	X-Ray Spine, Cerv (4 views)		□ 93017	ETT Tracing Only	
□ 90865	Counseling - Special Interview		□ 72090	X-Ray Spine; Scoliosis Ex		□ 93040	Electrocardiogram - Rhythm	
			□ 72110	Spine, lumbosacral; a/p & Lat		□ 96100	Psychological Testing	
IMMUNIZATIONS/INJECTIONS			□ 73030	Shoulder-Comp, min w/ 2vws		□ 99000	Specimen Handling	
□ 90585	BCG Vaccine		□ 73070	Elbow, anteropost & later vws		□ 99058	Office Emergency Care	
□ 90659	Influenza Virus Vaccine		□ 73120	X-Ray; Hand, 2 views		□ 99070	Surgical Tray - Misc.	
□ 90701	Immunization-DTP		□ 73560	X-Ray, Knee, 1 or 2 views		□ 99080	Special Reports of Med Rec	
□ 90702	DT Vaccine		□ 74022	X-Ray; Abdomen, Complete		□ 99195	Phlebotomy	
□ 90703	Tetanus Toxoids		□ 75552	Cardiac Magnetic Res Img		□		
□ 90732	Pneumococcal Vaccine		□ 76020	X-Ray; Bone Age Studies		□		
□ 90746	Hepatitis B Vaccine		□ 77054	Mammary Ductogram Complete		□		
□ 90749	Immunization: Unlisted		□ 78465	Myocardial Perfusion Img		□		

	ICD-9 CODE DIAGNOSIS		ICD-9 CODE DIAGNOSIS		ICD-9 CODE DIAGNOSIS
□ 009.0	Infect. colitis, enteritis, & gastroenteritis	□ 435.0	Basilar Artery Syndrome	□ 724.2	Pain: Lower Back
□ 133.0	Scabies	□ 440.0	Atherosclerosis	□ 727.67	Rupture of Achilles Tendon
□ 174.9	Breast Cancer, Female, Unspecified	□ 442.81	Carotid Artery	□ 780.1	Hallucinations
□ 185	Malignant neoplasm of prostate	□ 460	Common Cold (Acute Nasopharyngitis)	□ 780.3	Convulsions, Other
□ 250.00	Diabetes Mellitus w/o mention of Complication	□ 461.9	Acute Sinusitis	□ 780.50	Sleep Disturbances, Unspecified
□ 272.4	Hyperlipidemia	□ 474.00	Chronic Tonsillitis & Adenoiditis	□ 783.0	Anorexia
□ 282.5	Anemia, Sickle-cell Trait	□ 477.9	Allergic Rhinitis, Cause Unspecified	□ 783.1	Abnormal Weight Gain
□ 282.60	Sickle-cell disease, unspecified	□ 487.0	Influenza with pneumonia	□ 783.21	Abnormal Weight Loss
□ 285.9	Anemia, Unspecified	□ 496	Chronic Airway Obstruction	□ 823.80	Fractured Tibia
□ 300.4	Dysthymic disorder	□ 522.0	Pulpitis	□ 823.81	Fractured Fibula
□ 340	Multiple Sclerosis	□ 524.60	Temporo-Mandibular Joint Disorder - Unspec.	□ 831.00	Dislocated Shoulder, Closed, Unspecified
□ 342.90	Hemiplegia - Unspec.	□ 536.8	Stomach Pain	□ 835.00	Dislocated Hip, Closed, Unspecified
☒ 346.90	Migraine, unspecified	□ 553.3	Hiatal Hernia	□ 842.00	Sprained Wrist, Unspecified Site
□ 352.9	Unspecified disorder of cranial nerves	□ 564.1	Spastic Colon	□ 845.00	Sprained Ankle, Unspecified Site
□ 354.0	Carpal Tunnel Syndrome	□ 574.40	Chronic Hepatitis, Unspecified	□ 919.5	Insect Bite, Nonvenomous
□ 355.0	Sciatic Nerve Root Lesion	□ 571.5	Cirrhosis of Liver w/o mention of alcohol	□ 921.1	Contus Eyelid/Perioc Area
□ 366.9	Cataract	□ 573.3	Hepatitis	□ v16.3	Fam. Hist of Breast Cancer
□ 386.00	Menier's disease, unspecified	□ 575.2	Obstruction of Gallbladder	□ v17.4	Fam. Hist of Cardiovasc Dis
□ 401.1	Essential Hypertension, Benign	□ 648.20	Anemia - Compl. Pregnancy	□ v20.2	Well Child
□ 414.9	Ischemic Heart Disease	□ 715.90	Osteoarthritis - Unspec.	□ v22.0	Pregnancy - First Normal
□ 428.0	Congestive Heart Failure (CHF), unspecified	□ 721.3	Lumbar Osteo/Spondylarthrit	□ v22.1	Pregnancy - Normal

Previous Balance	Today's Charges	Total Due	Amount Paid	New Balance		Follow Up
					PRN _____ Weeks _____	Months _____ Units _____
_____	_____	_____	_____	_____	Next Appointment Date:	Time:

I hereby authorize release of any information acquired in the course of examination or treatment and allow a photocopy of my signature to be used.

_____

Figure 6-16 Procedure Entry – Carol Santos

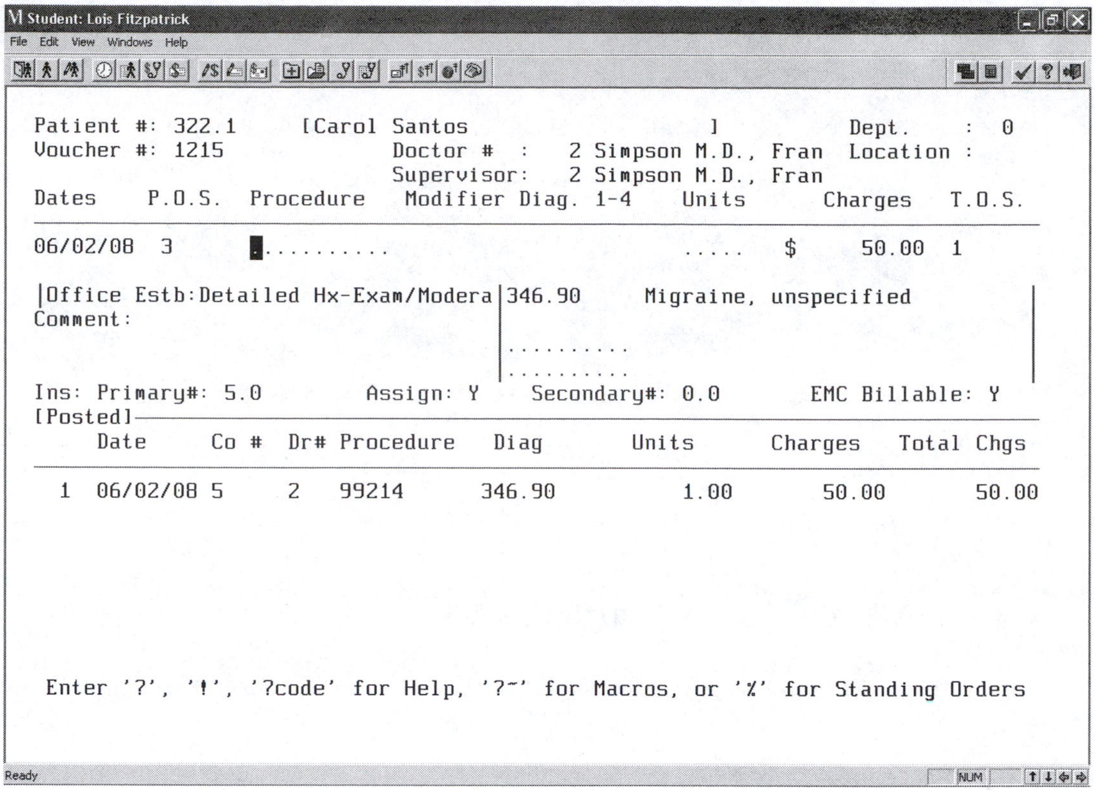

```
Ⅵ Student: Lois Fitzpatrick                                                    _ ⧉ ✕
File  Edit  View  Windows  Help

 Patient #: 322.1    [Carol Santos                    ]      Dept.   :  0
 Voucher #: 1215              Doctor # :   2 Simpson M.D., Fran  Location :
                             Supervisor:   2 Simpson M.D., Fran
 Dates    P.O.S.  Procedure   Modifier Diag. 1-4    Units      Charges  T.O.S.

 06/02/08  3      █.........                        .....   $    50.00  1

 |Office Estb:Detailed Hx-Exam/Modera|346.90    Migraine, unspecified
 Comment:                            |
                                     |    .........
                                     |    .........
 Ins: Primary#: 5.0        Assign: Y    Secondary#: 0.0      EMC Billable: Y
 [Posted]
      Date      Co #  Dr# Procedure   Diag      Units     Charges  Total Chgs

   1  06/02/08 5     2   99214     346.90       1.00      50.00      50.00




    Enter '?', '!', '?code' for Help, '?~' for Macros, or '%' for Standing Orders


Ready                                                          NUM    ↑↓↶↷
```

Since Carol Santos is giving a check for $16 (Figure 6-17), which includes her husband's visit copayment, you will need to go to the Payment Entry screen and apply the payment.

4. Apply the $16 check to the account by applying $8 to Paul's office visit and $8 to Carol's office visit. After you have applied the proper amount to both items, compare your screen to Figure 6-18.

Figure 6-17 Copayment from Paul and Carol Santos

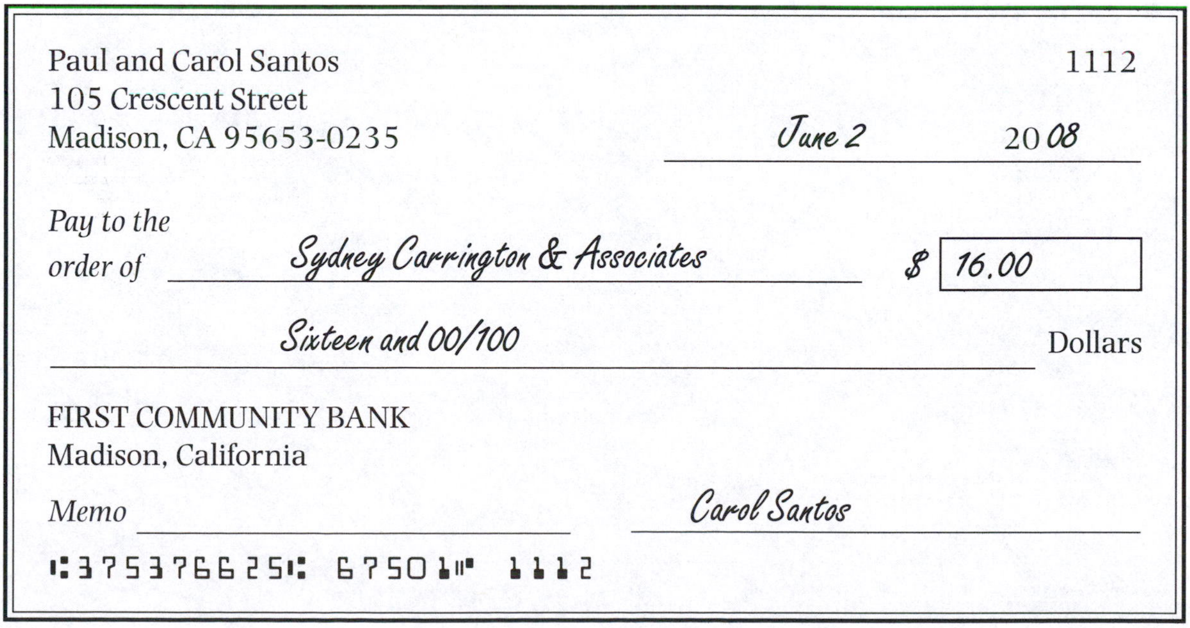

Paul and Carol Santos   1112
105 Crescent Street
Madison, CA 95653-0235   *June 2*   20 *08*

Pay to the
order of _____*Sydney Carrington & Associates*_____ $ | 16.00 |

            Sixteen and 00/100   Dollars

FIRST COMMUNITY BANK
Madison, California

Memo _____   *Carol Santos*

⑆375376625⑆ 6750⑈ 1112

Figure 6-18 Payment Screen After Copay Applied

```
M Student: Lois Fitzpatrick                                                    _ ☐ ☒
File  Edit  View  Windows  Help
☐☒ ☆ ☆☆ ☉ ☆☆☆ ☆☆☆ ☆☆ ☆☆ ☆☆ ☆☆☆ ☆☆☆☆                              ☒ ☒ ✓ ? ☆

   322-Santos, Paul R            Bal:    131.00 Pat Due:     0.00 Unappl:     0.00
   [Full]
    #   Serv Dt   Pat   Co#  Ins Bill  Dr ProCode  Adj Chgs  Receipts  Balance St

    1   06/02/08 Paul     5            2 99213       40.00     8.00    32.00 IU
    2   06/02/08 Paul     5            2 93000       57.00     0.00    57.00 IU
    3   06/02/08 Caro     5            2 99214       50.00     8.00    42.00 IU



   Type: (P)mt, (A)djust, (T)ransfer, (R)efund, (V)oid, (W)indow: █....... # : ..
   Source : (I)nsurance, (P)atient, (U)napplied, (O)ther        : .
   Ins Plan #: .....           Ref Date  : ......     Voucher : ........
   (C)heck, (M)oney, (O)ther: .                 Total Amount :$........

   Credit Line #, (U)napplied Credit, (A)uto range, (W)indow    : ........
   Doctor # to be Credited                                      : ...
   Approved  :$........  Visit Copay :$........
   Writedown :$........  Withholding :$........  Amount Credited :$........
   (S)ettle, (P)atient, (2)nd Ins, (B)illed 2nd, (R)ebill, (N)one: .      # : ..

      Batch: No Batch Selected    Pmts :$    16.00  Adj  :$      0.00
    (N)ext Page, (F)ormer Page, (B)atch, (C)heck, (\) to Repeat Last Entry :


Ready                                                            NUM    ↑↓↞↠
```

EXERCISE 5: USING AUTO PAY

STEPHEN WEILAND; ACCOUNT 323

GOAL(S): In this exercise, you will post charges and post a payment using automatic crediting.

1. Before posting your entry, study the encounter form in Figure 6-19. Answer the following questions:

   a. How many procedures were performed? _____

   b. What is the diagnosis? _____

   c. What is the total charge for this visit? _____

Figure 6-19   Encounter Form – Weiland

Sydney Carrington & Associates P.A.
34 Sycamore Street Suite 300
Madison, CA 95653

Date: 06/02/2008   Voucher No.: 1544

Time:

Patient: Stephen Weiland   Patient No: 323.1
Guarantor: Doctor: 3 – S. Carrington

CPT	DESCRIPTION	FEE	CPT	DESCRIPTION	FEE	CPT	DESCRIPTION	FEE
OFFICE/HOSPITAL CONSULTS			**LABORATORY/RADIOLOGY**			**PROCEDURES/TESTS**		
☐ 99201	Office New:Focused Hx-Exam		☒ 81000	Urinalysis	$8	☐ 00452	Anesthesia for Rad Surgery	
☐ 99202	Office New:Expanded Hx.Exam		☐ 81002	Urinalysis; Pregnancy Test		☐ 11100	Skin Biopsy	
☐ 99211	Office Estb:Min./None Hx-Exa		☐ 82951	Glucose Tolerance Test		☐ 15852	Dressing Change	
☐ 99212	Office Estb:Focused Hx-Exam		☐ 84478	Triglycerides		☐ 29075	Cast Appl. - Lower Arm	
☐ 99213	Office Estb:Expanded Hx-Exa		☐ 84550	Uric Acid: Blood Chemistry		☐ 29530	Strapping of Knee	
☒ 99214	Office Estb:Detailed Hx-Exa	$50	☐ 84830	Ovulation Test		☐ 29705	Removal/Revis of Cast w/Exa	
☐ 99215	Office Estb:Comprhn Hx-Exam		☒ 85014	Hematocrit	$18	☐ 53670	Catheterization Incl. Suppl	
☐ 99221	Hosp. Initial:Comprh Hx-		☐ 85032	Hemogram, Complete Blood Wk		☐ 57452	Colposcopy	
☐ 99223	Hosp. Ini:Comprh Hx-Exam/Hi		☐ 86403	Particle Agglutination Test		☐ 57505	ECC	
☐ 99231	Hosp. Subsequent: S-Fwd		☐ 86485	Skin Test; Candida		☐ 69420	Myringotomy	
☐ 99232	Hosp. Subsequent: Comprhn Hx		☐ 86580	TB Intradermal Test		☐ 92081	Visual Field Examination	
☐ 99233	Hosp. Subsequent: Ex/Hi		☐ 86585	TB Tine Test		☐ 92100	Serial Tonometry Exam	
☐ 99238	Hospital Visit Discharge Ex		☐ 87070	Culture		☐ 92120	Tonography	
☐ 99371	Telephone Consult - Simple		☐ 70190	X-Ray; Optic Foramina		☐ 92552	Pure Tone Audiometry	
☐ 99372	Telephone Consult - Intermed		☐ 70210	X-Ray Sinuses Complete		☐ 92567	Tympanometry	
☐ 99373	Telephone Consult - Complex		☐ 71010	Radiological Exam Ent Spine		☐ 93000	Electrocardiogram	
☐ 90840	Counseling - 25 minutes		☐ 71020	X-Ray Chest Pa & Lat		☐ 93015	Exercise Stress Test (ETT)	
☐ 90806	Counseling - 50 minutes		☐ 72050	X-Ray Spine, Cerv (4 views)		☐ 93017	ETT Tracing Only	
☐ 90865	Counseling - Special Interview		☐ 72090	X-Ray Spine; Scoliosis Ex		☐ 93040	Electrocardiogram - Rhythm	
			☐ 72110	Spine, lumbosacral; a/p & Lat		☐ 96100	Psychological Testing	
IMMUNIZATIONS/INJECTIONS			☐ 73030	Shoulder-Comp, min w/ 2vws		☐ 99000	Specimen Handling	
☐ 90585	BCG Vaccine		☐ 73070	Elbow, anteropost & later vws		☐ 99058	Office Emergency Care	
☐ 90659	Influenza Virus Vaccine		☐ 73120	X-Ray; Hand, 2 views		☐ 99070	Surgical Tray - Misc.	
☐ 90701	Immunization-DTP		☐ 73560	X-Ray, Knee, 1 or 2 views		☐ 99080	Special Reports of Med Rec	
☐ 90702	DT Vaccine		☐ 74022	X-Ray; Abdomen, Complete		☐ 99195	Phlebotomy	
☐ 90703	Tetanus Toxoids		☐ 75552	Cardiac Magnetic Res Img		☐		
☐ 90732	Pneumococcal Vaccine		☐ 76020	X-Ray; Bone Age Studies		☐		
☐ 90746	Hepatitis B Vaccine		☐ 77054	Mammary Ductogram Complete		☐		
☒ 90749	Immunization: Unlisted	$12	☐ 78465	Myocardial Perfusion Img		☐		

ICD-9 CODE DIAGNOSIS			ICD-9 CODE DIAGNOSIS			ICD-9 CODE DIAGNOSIS	
☐ 009.0	Infect. colitis, enteritis, & gastroenteritis		☐ 435.0	Basilar Artery Syndrome		☐ 724.2	Pain: Lower Back
☐ 133.0	Scabies		☐ 440.0	Atherosclerosis		☐ 727.67	Rupture of Achilles Tendon
☐ 174.9	Breast Cancer, Female, Unspecified		☐ 442.81	Carotid Artery		☐ 780.1	Hallucinations
☐ 185	Malignant neoplasm of prostate		☐ 460	Common Cold (Acute Nasopharyngitis)		☐ 780.3	Convulsions, Other
☐ 250.00	Diabetes Mellitus w/o mention of Complication		☐ 461.9	Acute Sinusitis		☐ 780.50	Sleep Disturbances, Unspecified
☐ 272.4	Hyperlipidemia		☐ 474.00	Chronic Tonsillitis & Adenoiditis		☐ 783.0	Anorexia
☐ 282.5	Anemia, Sickle-cell Trait		☐ 477.9	Allergic Rhinitis, Cause Unspecified		☐ 783.1	Abnormal Weight Gain
☐ 282.60	Sickle-cell disease, unspecified		☐ 487.0	Influenza with pneumonia		☐ 783.21	Abnormal Weight Loss
☐ 285.9	Anemia, Unspecified		☐ 496	Chronic Airway Obstruction		☐ 823.80	Fractured Tibia
☐ 300.4	Dysthymic disorder		☐ 522.0	Pulpitis		☐ 823.81	Fractured Fibula
☐ 340	Multiple Sclerosis		☐ 524.60	Temporo-Mandibular Joint Disorder - Unspec.		☐ 831.00	Dislocated Shoulder, Closed, Unspecified
☐ 342.90	Hemiplegia - Unspec.		☐ 536.8	Stomach Pain		☐ 835.00	Dislocated Hip, Closed, Unspecified
☐ 346.90	Migraine, unspecified		☐ 553.3	Hiatal Hernia		☐ 842.00	Sprained Wrist, Unspecified Site
☐ 352.9	Unspecified disorder of cranial nerves		☐ 564.1	Spastic Colon		☐ 845.00	Sprained Ankle, Unspecified Site
☐ 354.0	Carpal Tunnel Syndrome		☐ 574.40	Chronic Hepatitis, Unspecified		☐ 919.5	Insect Bite, Nonvenomous
☐ 355.0	Sciatic Nerve Root Lesion		☐ 571.5	Cirrhosis of Liver w/o mention of alcohol		☐ 921.1	Contus Eyelid/Perioc Area
☐ 366.9	Cataract		☐ 573.3	Hepatitis		☐ v16.3	Fam. Hist of Breast Cancer
☐ 386.00	Menier's disease, unspecified		☐ 575.2	Obstruction of Gallbladder		☐ v17.4	Fam. Hist of Cardiovasc Dis
☐ 401.1	Essential Hypertension, Benign		☐ 648.20	Anemia - Compl. Pregnancy		☒ v20.2	Well Child
☐ 414.9	Ischemic Heart Disease		☐ 715.90	Osteoarthritis - Unspec.		☐ v22.0	Pregnancy - First Normal
☐ 428.0	Congestive Heart Failure (CHF), unspecified		☐ 721.3	Lumbar Osteo/Spondylarthrit		☐ v22.1	Pregnancy - Normal

Previous Balance	Today's Charges	Total Due	Amount Paid	New Balance		Follow Up
_____	_____	_____	$88 check #427		PRN _____ Weeks _____	Months _____ Units _____
					Next Appointment Date:	Time:

I hereby authorize release of any information acquired in the course of
examination or treatment and allow a photocopy of my signature to be used.

_____

2. Based on the information found on the encounter form, post the charges for Stephen Weiland. After you have posted the charges, compare your screen to Figure 6-20.

3. Post the payment (Figure 6-21) from the Payment Entry screen, using the automatic crediting feature. Compare your screen to Figure 6-22 before you press the F1 key. Compare your screen to Figure 6-23 after you have pressed the F1 key.

Figure 6-20 Four Procedures Posted – Weiland

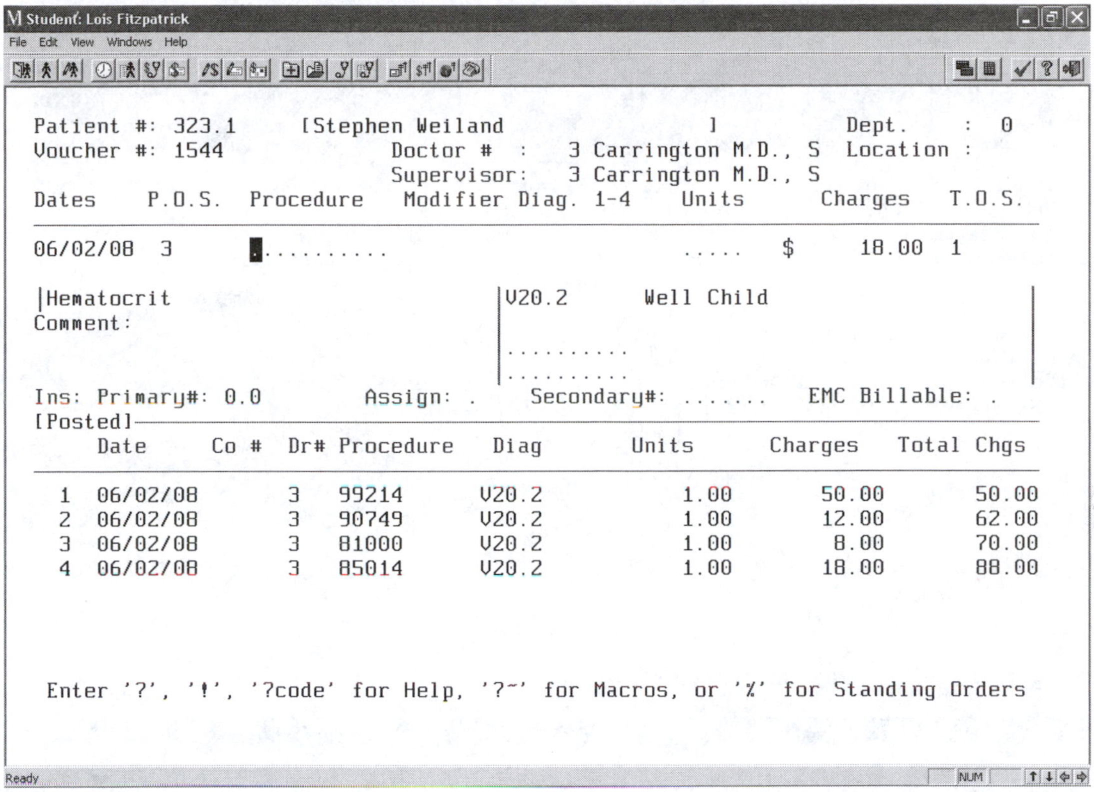

```
Student: Lois Fitzpatrick
File  Edit  View  Windows  Help

Patient #: 323.1      [Stephen Weiland              ]          Dept.     :  0
Voucher #: 1544                 Doctor #   :    3 Carrington M.D., S  Location :
                                Supervisor:     3 Carrington M.D., S
Dates      P.O.S.  Procedure    Modifier Diag. 1-4    Units       Charges    T.O.S.

06/02/08   3       ..........                        .....   $      18.00   1

|Hematocrit                           |V20.2      Well Child
Comment:                              |
                                      |..........
                                      |..........
Ins: Primary#: 0.0        Assign: .    Secondary#: .......     EMC Billable: .
[Posted]
     Date        Co #   Dr# Procedure    Diag         Units        Charges    Total Chgs

  1  06/02/08           3   99214        V20.2         1.00          50.00         50.00
  2  06/02/08           3   90749        V20.2         1.00          12.00         62.00
  3  06/02/08           3   81000        V20.2         1.00           8.00         70.00
  4  06/02/08           3   85014        V20.2         1.00          18.00         88.00

 Enter '?', '!', '?code' for Help, '?~' for Macros, or '%' for Standing Orders

Ready                                                                    NUM
```

Figure 6-21 Check from Patient – Weiland

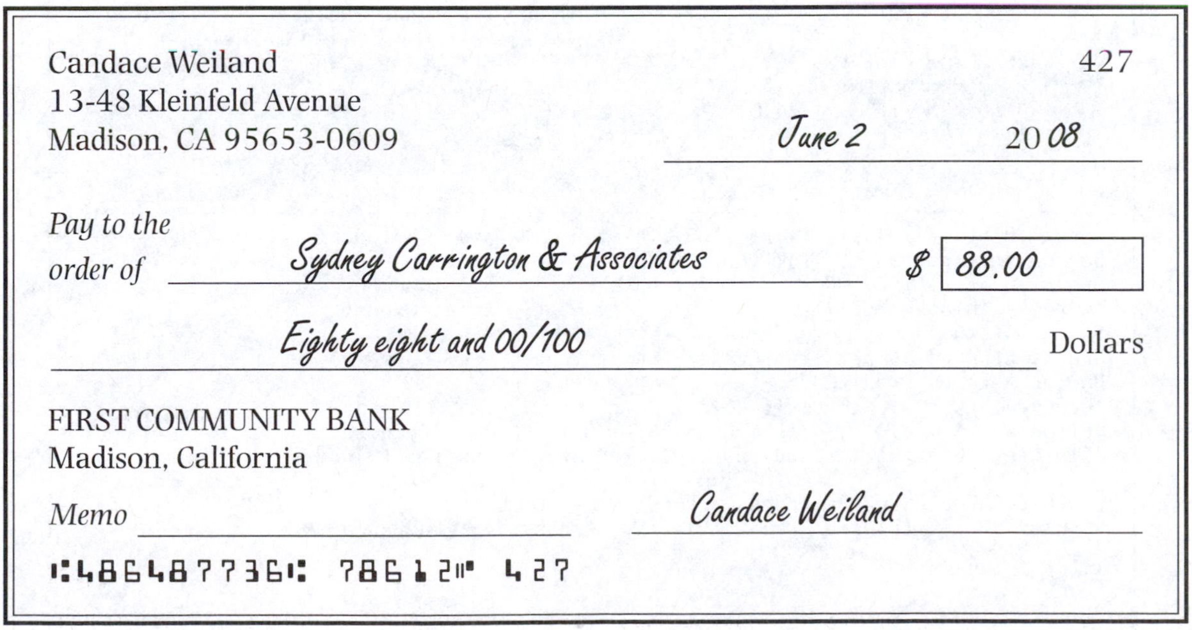

Candace Weiland 427
13-48 Kleinfeld Avenue
Madison, CA 95653-0609 June 2 20 08

Pay to the order of Sydney Carrington & Associates $ 88.00

Eighty eight and 00/100 Dollars

FIRST COMMUNITY BANK
Madison, California

Memo Candace Weiland

⑆486487736⑆ 78612⑈ 427

Figure 6-22 Payment Screen Before Posting

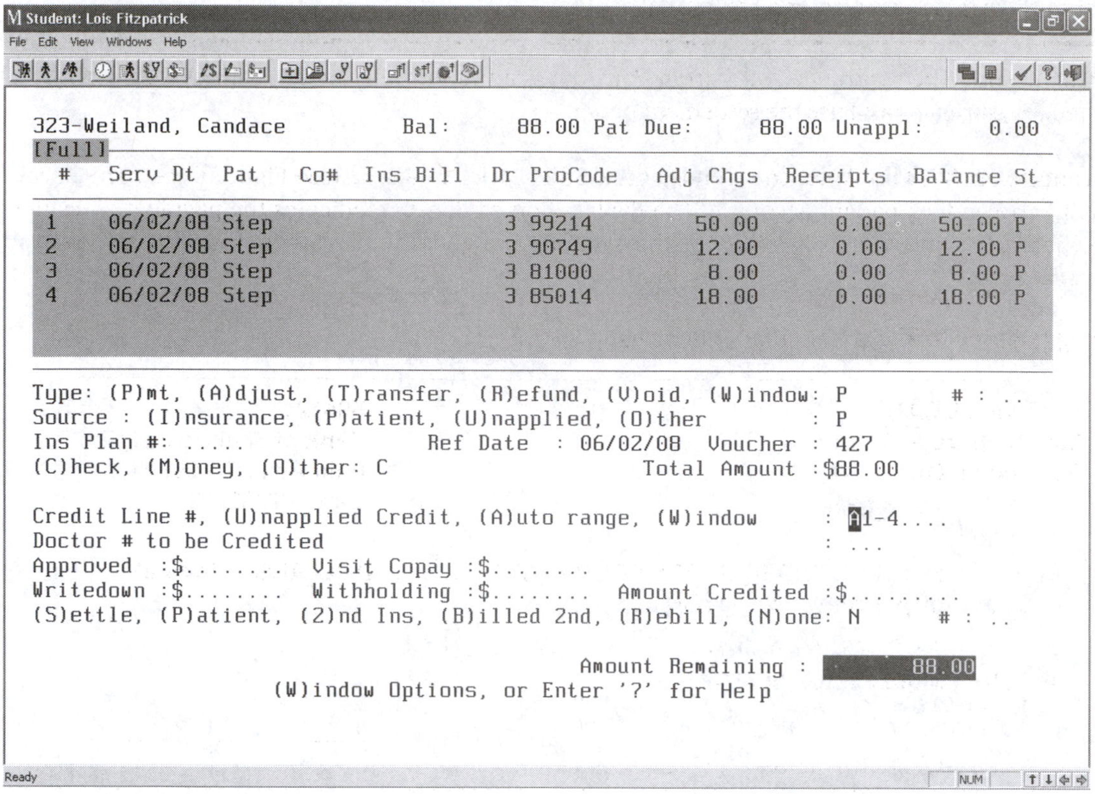

Figure 6-23 Payment Screen After Posting

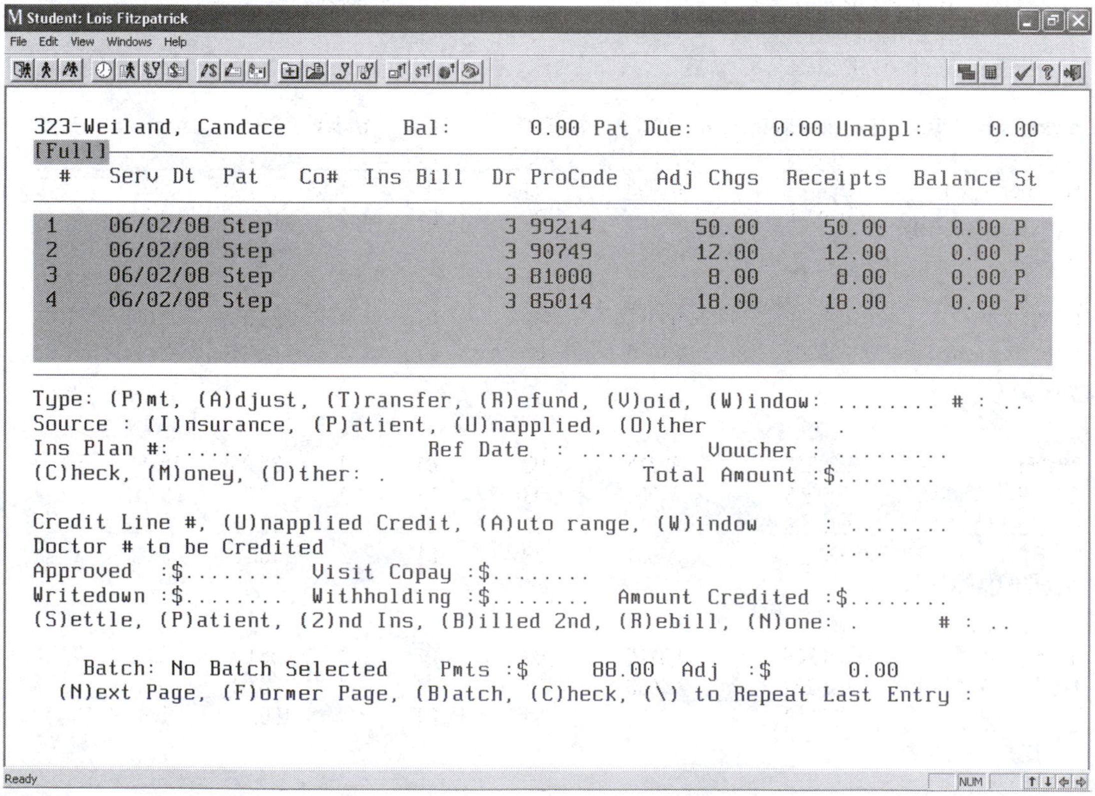

EXERCISE 6: POSTING INSURANCE PAYMENT SPLIT BETWEEN PATIENTS

GOAL(S): Apply the insurance check from Pan American to four different patient accounts. You will bill secondary insurances and use the settlement option.

Insurance plan #7, Pan American, sends check 584121 for $444.82 (see Figure 6-24). The check is to be split between four patient accounts. The Explanation of Benefits indicates the payment allocations for each charge. In some cases, you will settle the remaining balances, and in others you will bill the secondary insurance plan.

Figure 6-24 Explanation of Benefits

PAN AMERICAN	584121
259 Anchorage Avenue	Bank of America
San Diego, CA 96588	Palo Alto, CA 96344
	Date: 06/02/08

PAY   **FOUR HUNDRED FORTY FOUR AND 82/100.......DOLLARS $444.82**

TO   **SYDNEY CARRINGTON, MD**

THE   **34 Sycamore Street**

ORDER   **Madison,CA 95653**

OF

100911199 08 324411778: 03

06/02/08

Pan American Insurance Company
Explanation of Benefits

Provider: Sydney Carrington, MD   Provider #: 1155123
             34 Sycamore Street
             Madison, CA 95653

ID/Patient	Service Date	CPT	POS	TOS	Units	Chg	Copay	Paid
463127934	020208	99214	03	01	1	50.00	10.00	32.48
Hatcher, Craig	020208	81000	03	01	1	8.00	0.00	6.23
	020208	85031	03	01	1	15.00	0.00	12.64
							Total	51.35
PX671352	020208	99215	03	01	1	85.00	8.00	70.45
Roberts, Ashleigh	020208	81000	03	01	1	8.00	0.00	6.23
							Total	76.68
781356	020208	99215	03	01	1	85.00	15.00	59.72
Scheller, Denise	020208	81000	03	01	1	8.00	0.00	6.23
	020208	85014	03	01	1	18.00	0.00	16.84
	020208	85031	03	01	1	15.00	0.00	12.64
							Total	95.43
461461461	020208	99215	03	01	1	85.00	2.00	76.34
Fitzpatrick, Mark	020208	81000	03	01	1	8.00	0.00	6.23
	020208	72050	03	01	1	150.00	0.00	138.79
							Total	221.36

NOTE: *After choosing to settle or bill the secondary insurance plan, you will be warned that the item is pending insurance billing. For the purposes of this exercise, choose "Y" to continue.*

1. Before posting your entry, study the explanation of benefits in Figure 6-24. Answer the following questions.

    a. What patient accounts are being paid by Pan American? _____

    b. What are the total payments for each account? _____

    c. What are the service dates that are being paid by Pan American? _____

2. Based on the information found on the explanation of benefits, post the payments for each patient separately. Enter the total paid for each patient as the amount of the check for that patient. Apply the amounts for each line exactly as shown. For each patient, compare your screen to the figure before posting the first payment and the figure after the successful posting of all items for that patient.

Figure 6-25 Before Posting First Item – Hatcher

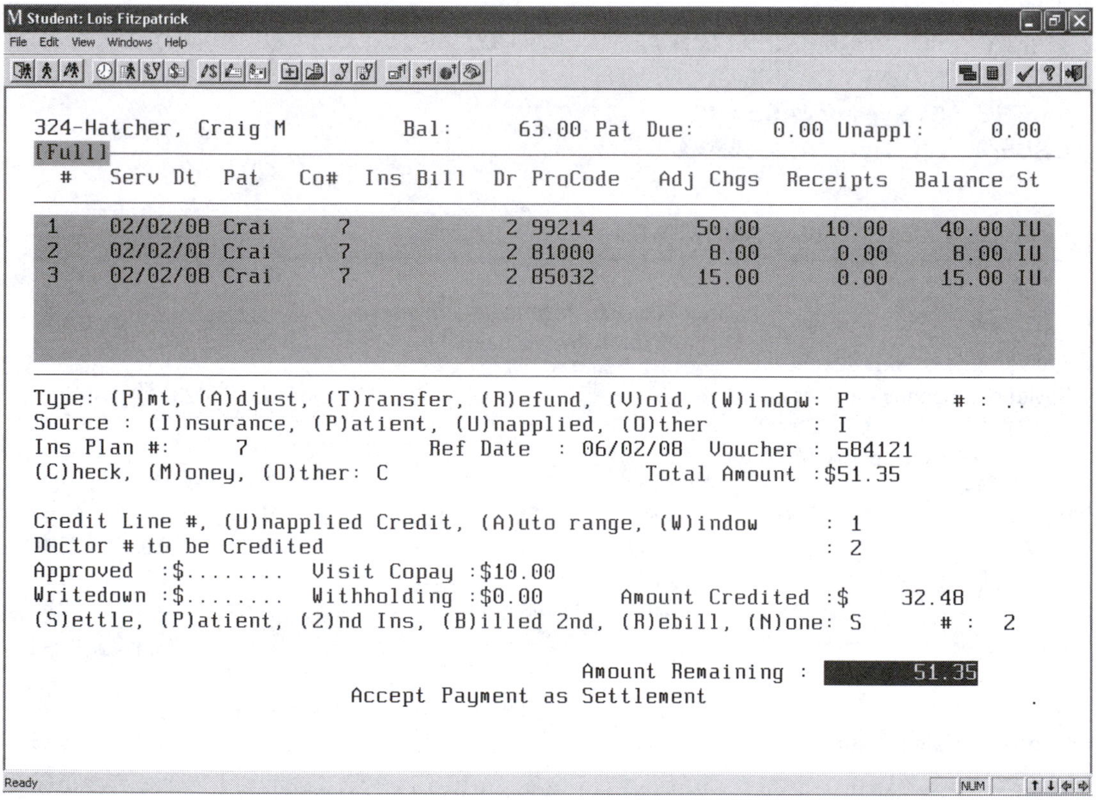

Figure 6-26 After Posting Last Item – Hatcher

```
M Student: Lois Fitzpatrick                                                    _ ☐ ✕
File  Edit  View  Windows  Help
🔲🔲🔲 🔲🔲🔲🔲 🔲🔲🔲 🔲🔲🔲🔲 🔲🔲🔲🔲                                    🔲🔲 ✓ ? 🔲

  324-Hatcher, Craig M          Bal:     0.00 Pat Due:     0.00 Unappl:     0.00
 [Full]
    #   Serv Dt  Pat   Co#  Ins Bill  Dr ProCode  Adj Chgs  Receipts  Balance  St

    1   02/02/08 Crai    7          2 99214       42.48i    42.48     0.00 IU
    2   02/02/08 Crai    7          2 81000        6.23i     6.23     0.00 IU
    3   02/02/08 Crai    7          2 85032       12.64i    12.64     0.00 IU




  Type: (P)mt, (A)djust, (T)ransfer, (R)efund, (V)oid, (W)indow: █.......  # : ..
  Source : (I)nsurance, (P)atient, (U)napplied, (O)ther         : .
  Ins Plan #:  .....        Ref Date  : ......     Voucher  : ........
  (C)heck, (M)oney, (O)ther: .              Total Amount :$.......

  Credit Line #, (U)napplied Credit, (A)uto range, (W)indow     : ........
  Doctor # to be Credited                                       : ...
  Approved  :$.......  Visit Copay :$........
  Writedown :$.......  Withholding :$........  Amount Credited :$.......
  (S)ettle, (P)atient, (2)nd Ins, (B)illed 2nd, (R)ebill, (N)one: .   # : ..

        Batch: No Batch Selected     Pmts :$    51.35  Adj  :$    11.65
     (N)ext Page, (F)ormer Page, (B)atch, (C)heck, (\) to Repeat Last Entry :


Ready                                                          NUM    ↑↓⇦⇨
```

Figure 6-27 Before Posting First Item – Roberts

```
M Student: Lois Fitzpatrick                                                    _ ☐ ✕
File  Edit  View  Windows  Help
🔲🔲🔲 🔲🔲🔲🔲 🔲🔲🔲 🔲🔲🔲🔲 🔲🔲🔲🔲                                    🔲🔲 ✓ ? 🔲

  325-Roberts, Ashleigh K        Bal:    85.00 Pat Due:     0.00 Unappl:     0.00
 [Full]
    #   Serv Dt  Pat   Co#  Ins Bill  Dr ProCode  Adj Chgs  Receipts  Balance  St

    1   02/02/08 Ashl    7          1 99215       85.00      8.00    77.00 IU
    2   02/02/08 Ashl    7          1 81000        8.00      0.00     8.00 IU




  Type: (P)mt, (A)djust, (T)ransfer, (R)efund, (V)oid, (W)indow: P        # : ..
  Source : (I)nsurance, (P)atient, (U)napplied, (O)ther         : I
  Ins Plan #:      7          Ref Date  : 06/02/08  Voucher  : 584121
  (C)heck, (M)oney, (O)ther: C              Total Amount :$76.68

  Credit Line #, (U)napplied Credit, (A)uto range, (W)indow     : 1
  Doctor # to be Credited                                       : 1
  Approved  :$.......  Visit Copay :$8.00
  Writedown :$.......  Withholding :$0.00   Amount Credited :$   70.45
  (S)ettle, (P)atient, (2)nd Ins, (B)illed 2nd, (R)ebill, (N)one: S   # :  2

                                 Amount Remaining  :         76.68
                       Accept Payment as Settlement                        .


Ready                                                          NUM    ↑↓⇦⇨
```

Figure 6-28 After Posting Last Item – Roberts

```
M Student: Lois Fitzpatrick                                              _ ▯ X
File  Edit  View  Windows  Help

[toolbar icons]                                                  [toolbar icons]

  325-Roberts, Ashleigh K       Bal:      0.00 Pat Due:      0.00 Unappl:     0.00
  [Full]
   #   Serv Dt   Pat   Co#  Ins Bill  Dr ProCode   Adj Chgs  Receipts  Balance St

   1   02/02/08 Ashl    7               1 99215      78.45i    78.45     0.00 IU
   2   02/02/08 Ashl    7               1 81000       6.23i     6.23     0.00 IU



  Type: (P)mt, (A)djust, (T)ransfer, (R)efund, (V)oid, (W)indow: ........ # : ..
  Source : (I)nsurance, (P)atient, (U)napplied, (O)ther        : .
  Ins Plan #: .....            Ref Date  : ......      Voucher : ........
  (C)heck, (M)oney, (O)ther: .                   Total Amount :$........

  Credit Line #, (U)napplied Credit, (A)uto range, (W)indow    : ........
  Doctor # to be Credited                                      : ...
  Approved  :$........  Visit Copay :$........
  Writedown :$........  Withholding :$........  Amount Credited :$........
  (S)ettle, (P)atient, (2)nd Ins, (B)illed 2nd, (R)ebill, (N)one: .      # : ..

     Batch: No Batch Selected     Pmts :$    128.03  Adj  :$     19.97
     (N)ext Page, (F)ormer Page, (B)atch, (C)heck, (\) to Repeat Last Entry :

New Patient                                                       NUM   ↑↓⇐⇒
```

Figure 6-29 Before Posting First Item – Scheller

```
M Student: Lois Fitzpatrick                                              _ ▯ X
File  Edit  View  Windows  Help

[toolbar icons]                                                  [toolbar icons]

  326-Scheller, Denise L        Bal:    111.00 Pat Due:      0.00 Unappl:     0.00
  [Full]
   #   Serv Dt   Pat   Co#  Ins Bill  Dr ProCode   Adj Chgs  Receipts  Balance St

   1   02/02/08 Deni    7'              3 99215      85.00     15.00    70.00 IU
   2   02/02/08 Deni    7'              3 81000       8.00      0.00     8.00 IU
   3   02/02/08 Deni    7'              3 85014      18.00      0.00    18.00 IU
   4   02/02/08 Deni    7'              3 85032      15.00      0.00    15.00 IU


  Type: (P)mt, (A)djust, (T)ransfer, (R)efund, (V)oid, (W)indow: P        # : ..
  Source : (I)nsurance, (P)atient, (U)napplied, (O)ther        : I
  Ins Plan #:     7            Ref Date  : 06/02/08  Voucher : 584121
  (C)heck, (M)oney, (O)ther: C                   Total Amount :$95.43

  Credit Line #, (U)napplied Credit, (A)uto range, (W)indow    : 1......
  Doctor # to be Credited                                      : 3
  Approved  :$........  Visit Copay :$15.00
  Writedown :$........  Withholding :$0.00   Amount Credited :$    59.72
  (S)ettle, (P)atient, (2)nd Ins, (B)illed 2nd, (R)ebill, (N)one: 2     # : ..
  Ins Plan#: 11.0

                              Amount Remaining :        95.43
               (W)indow Options, or Enter '?' for Help

Ready                                                             NUM   ↑↓⇐⇒
```

Figure 6-30   After Posting Last Item – Scheller

```
M Student: Lois Fitzpatrick                                                    [_][8][X]
File  Edit  View  Windows  Help

[toolbar icons]                                                    [icons]  √ ? 

  326-Scheller, Denise L      Bal:      15.57 Pat Due:      0.00 Unappl:      0.00
  [Full]
    #   Serv Dt  Pat   Co#  Ins Bill  Dr ProCode   Adj Chgs  Receipts  Balance St

    1    02/02/08 Deni   11           3 99215      85.00i    74.72    10.28 IU
    2    02/02/08 Deni   11           3 81000       8.00i     6.23     1.77 IU
    3    02/02/08 Deni   11           3 85014      18.00i    16.84     1.16 IU
    4    02/02/08 Deni   11           3 85032      15.00i    12.64     2.36 IU


  Type: (P)mt, (A)djust, (T)ransfer, (R)efund, (V)oid, (W)indow: ▮.......  # : ..
  Source : (I)nsurance, (P)atient, (U)napplied, (O)ther        : .
  Ins Plan #: .....            Ref Date  : ......    Voucher : .
  (C)heck, (M)oney, (O)ther: .                Total Amount :$.......

  Credit Line #, (U)napplied Credit, (A)uto range, (W)indow     : ........
  Doctor # to be Credited                                       : ...
  Approved  :$....... Visit Copay :$.......
  Writedown :$....... Withholding :$....... Amount Credited :$.......
  (S)ettle, (P)atient, (2)nd Ins, (B)illed 2nd, (R)ebill, (N)one: .    # : ..

      Batch: No Batch Selected    Pmts :$   223.46 Adj  :$    19.97
   (N)ext Page, (F)ormer Page, (B)atch, (C)heck, (\) to Repeat Last Entry :


Ready                                                          NUM   ↑↓⇦⇨
```

Figure 6-31   Before Posting First Item – Fitzpatrick

```
M Student: Lois Fitzpatrick                                                    [_][8][X]
File  Edit  View  Windows  Help

[toolbar icons]                                                    [icons]  √ ? 

  327-Fitzpatrick, Mark P      Bal:     241.00 Pat Due:      0.00 Unappl:      0.00
  [Full]
    #   Serv Dt  Pat   Co#  Ins Bill  Dr ProCode   Adj Chgs  Receipts  Balance St

    1    02/02/08 Mark    7          1 99215      85.00      2.00    83.00 IU
    2    02/02/08 Mark    7          1 81000       8.00      0.00     8.00 IU
    3    02/02/08 Mark    7          1 72050     150.00      0.00   150.00 IU


  Type: (P)mt, (A)djust, (T)ransfer, (R)efund, (V)oid, (W)indow: P       # : ..
  Source : (I)nsurance, (P)atient, (U)napplied, (O)ther        : I
  Ins Plan #:      7           Ref Date  : 06/02/08  Voucher : 584121
  (C)heck, (M)oney, (O)ther: C                Total Amount :$221.36

  Credit Line #, (U)napplied Credit, (A)uto range, (W)indow     : 1
  Doctor # to be Credited                                       : 1
  Approved  :$....... Visit Copay :$2.00
  Writedown :$....... Withholding :$0.00  Amount Credited :$   76.34
  (S)ettle, (P)atient, (2)nd Ins, (B)illed 2nd, (R)ebill, (N)one: S    # :  2

                                Amount Remaining :      221.36
                   Accept Payment as Settlement                       ▮


Ready                                                          NUM   ↑↓⇦⇨
```

Figure 6-32   After Posting Last Item – Fitzpatrick

```
M Student: Lois Fitzpatrick                                          _ ⊡ ☒
File  Edit  View  Windows  Help

[toolbar icons]                                              [toolbar icons]

 327-Fitzpatrick, Mark P      Bal:     0.00 Pat Due:    0.00 Unappl:     0.00
[Full]
  #   Serv Dt   Pat    Co#  Ins Bill  Dr ProCode   Adj Chgs  Receipts  Balance St

  1   02/02/08 Mark    7              1 99215        78.34i    78.34     0.00 IU
  2   02/02/08 Mark    7              1 81000         6.23i     6.23     0.00 IU
  3   02/02/08 Mark    7              1 72050       138.79i   138.79     0.00 IU


Type: (P)mt, (A)djust, (T)ransfer, (R)efund, (V)oid, (W)indow: ▮....... # : ..
Source : (I)nsurance, (P)atient, (U)napplied, (O)ther       : .
Ins Plan #: .....          Ref Date   : ......      Voucher : ........
(C)heck, (M)oney, (O)ther: .                  Total Amount :$.......

Credit Line #, (U)napplied Credit, (A)uto range, (W)indow    : ........
Doctor # to be Credited                                      : ...
Approved  :$........  Visit Copay :$........
Writedown :$........  Withholding :$........  Amount Credited :$.......
(S)ettle, (P)atient, (2)nd Ins, (B)illed 2nd, (R)ebill, (N)one: .      # : ..

   Batch: No Batch Selected      Pmts :$    444.82  Adj  :$     39.61
   (N)ext Page, (F)ormer Page, (B)atch, (C)heck, (\) to Repeat Last Entry :


Ready                                                          NUM   ↑↓⇐⇒
```

U N I T 7

Report
Generation

In the unit exercises that follow, you will generate a Guarantors' Financial Summary report, Current Period report, and System Financial Summary report and print patient statements.

NOTE: The reports will be based on the account activity entered to date. Therefore, the report information will vary by the unit exercises that have been completed.

EXERCISE 1: GUARANTORS' FINANCIAL SUMMARY

GOAL(S): In this exercise, you will generate a Guarantors' Financial Summary report.

1. Generate the Guarantors' Financial Summary Report based on the following information:

   a. Send the report to the printer.

   b. Generate the report by account number for all accounts.

   c. Accept the default answers for the remaining fields.

   d. Compare your screen to Figure 7-1, Guarantors' Financial Summary Report Selection Screen, and press F1 to print the report (Figure 7-2).

129

Figure 7-1 Guarantors' Financial Summary Report Selection Screen

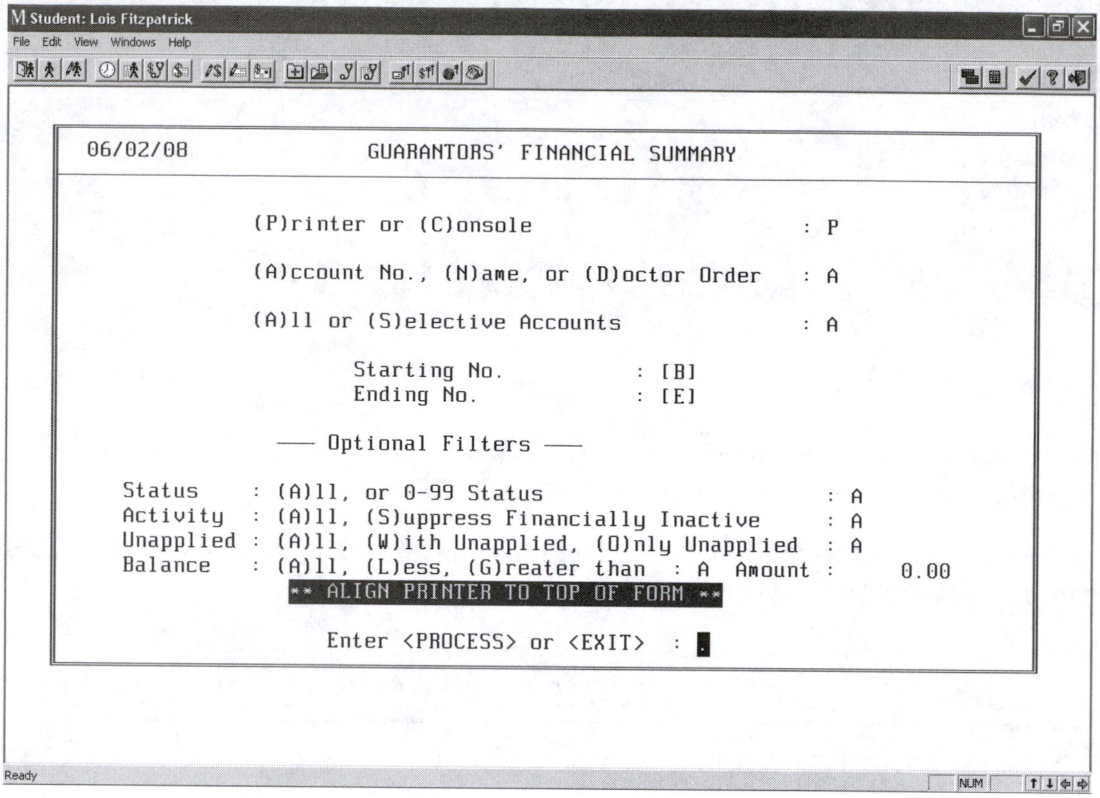

```
M Student: Lois Fitzpatrick                                                    _ □ ×
File  Edit  View  Windows  Help

▣▯▯ ▯▯▯ ▯▯▯ ▯▯▯ ▯▯ ▯▯▯ ▯▯▯ ▯▯▯ ▯                                        ▯▯ ✓ ? ▯

┌──────────────────────────────────────────────────────────────────────┐
│  06/02/08                    GUARANTORS' FINANCIAL SUMMARY             │
│                                                                        │
│               (P)rinter or (C)onsole                      : P         │
│                                                                        │
│               (A)ccount No., (N)ame, or (D)octor Order    : A         │
│                                                                        │
│               (A)ll or (S)elective Accounts               : A         │
│                                                                        │
│                    Starting No.        : [B]                          │
│                    Ending No.          : [E]                          │
│                                                                        │
│                    ──── Optional Filters ────                         │
│                                                                        │
│      Status   : (A)ll, or 0-99 Status                     : A         │
│      Activity : (A)ll, (S)uppress Financially Inactive    : A         │
│      Unapplied: (A)ll, (W)ith Unapplied, (O)nly Unapplied : A         │
│      Balance  : (A)ll, (L)ess, (G)reater than  : A  Amount :   0.00   │
│              ** ALIGN PRINTER TO TOP OF FORM **                       │
│                                                                        │
│               Enter <PROCESS> or <EXIT>  : ▮                          │
│                                                                        │
└──────────────────────────────────────────────────────────────────────┘

Ready                                                          NUM     ↑↓←→
```

Figure 7-2 Guarantors' Financial Summary Report

```
06/02/08                        GUARANTORS' FINANCIAL SUMMARY BY ACCOUNT                      Page 1
                                     Student: Lois Fitzpatrick
                                          All Accounts
                                         Status : ALL

Accnt #   Last Name          -Last Statement Data-  --Last Payment Data--  YTD Chgs  Unappl Cr  Pat Due AR  Balance
=================================================================================================================
300       Walters, Charles           0.00                       0.00         0.00      0.00        0.00       0.00
301       Rojas, Yvonne              0.00                       0.00         0.00      0.00        0.00       0.00
302       Glenmore, Edward           0.00                       0.00         0.00      0.00        0.00       0.00
303       Monaco, Anthony            0.00                       0.00         0.00      0.00        0.00       0.00
304       Monti, Vincent             0.00                       0.00         0.00      0.00        0.00       0.00
305       Viajo, Catherine           0.00                       0.00        40.00      0.00        0.00      40.00
306       Cusack, Christine          0.00                       0.00        98.00      0.00        0.00      98.00
307       Wyatt, John                0.00                       0.00        73.00      0.00        0.00      73.00
308       Frost, William             0.00                       0.00         0.00      0.00        0.00       0.00
309       Perez, Juan                0.00                       0.00        50.00      0.00       50.00      50.00
310       Stanch, Rebecca            0.00                       0.00       160.00      0.00        0.00     160.00
311       Vega, Roberto              0.00                       0.00       200.00      0.00        0.00     200.00
312       Salvani, William           0.00                       0.00         0.00      0.00        0.00       0.00
313       Stein, Erin                0.00                       0.00         0.00      0.00        0.00       0.00
314       Fuentas, Carman            0.00                       0.00         0.00      0.00        0.00       0.00
315       Morgan, Margaret           0.00                       0.00       126.00      0.00        0.00     126.00
316       Barker, Sharon             0.00                       0.00        89.00      0.00        0.00      89.00
317       Lopez, Sonia               0.00                       0.00        55.00      0.00        0.00      55.00
318       Brinkman, Gary             0.00                       0.00       418.00      0.00        0.00     418.00
319       Miles, Wayne               0.00  06/02/08           123.00       123.00      0.00        0.00       0.00
320       Ramirez, Leanna            0.00  06/02/08            10.00        55.00      0.00        0.00      45.00
321       Marchese, Anna             0.00  06/02/08            40.00        40.00      0.00        0.00       0.00
322       Santos, Paul               0.00  06/02/08            16.00       147.00      0.00        0.00     131.00
323       Weiland, Candace           0.00  06/02/08            88.00        88.00      0.00        0.00       0.00
324       Hatcher, Craig             0.00  06/02/08            51.35        61.35      0.00        0.00       0.00
325       Roberts, Ashleigh          0.00  06/02/08            76.68        84.68      0.00        0.00       0.00
326       Scheller, Denise           0.00  06/02/08            95.43       126.00      0.00        0.00      15.57
327       Fitzpatrick, Mark          0.00  06/02/08           221.36       223.36      0.00        0.00       0.00
328       Penny, Robert              0.00  02/16/08           130.00       111.00     19.00      -19.00     -19.00
329       Knifert, John              0.00  02/16/08            63.00        71.00      0.00        0.00      63.00
330       Zapola, Karen              0.00  02/16/08           155.00       155.00      0.00        0.00       0.00
331       Jones, Elizabeth           0.00  02/16/08             5.00        65.00      0.00        0.00      60.00
332       Walker, Ross               0.00                       0.00         0.00      0.00        0.00       0.00
333       Swindel, Alan              0.00                       0.00         0.00      0.00        0.00       0.00
334       Berntson, Allison          0.00                       0.00         0.00      0.00        0.00       0.00
335       Cantorelli, Brittany       0.00                       0.00         0.00      0.00        0.00       0.00
336       Valentine, Michael         0.00                       0.00         0.00      0.00        0.00       0.00
=================================================================================================================

          TOTALS :                                                       2,659.39     19.00       31.00   1,604.57


                           ****  Number Printed : 37   ****
                           ****  Number Active  : 37   ****
```

NOTE: *The reports will be based on the account activity entered to date. Therefore, the report information will vary by the unit exercises that have been completed.*

EXERCISE 2: CURRENT PERIOD REPORT

GOAL(S): In this exercise, you will generate a Current Period Report.

1. Generate the Current Period Report based on the following information:

   a. Generate the report based on summary information.

   b. Generate the report for the period to date, for all accounts.

   c. Compare your screen to Figure 7-3, then press F1 to print the report (Figure 7-4).

Figure 7-3 Current Period Report Selection Screen

```
M Student: Lois Fitzpatrick                                     _ □ X
File  Edit  View  Windows  Help



   06/02/08                      CURRENT PERIOD REPORT



                 (D)etail or (S)ummary                    : S

                 (P)eriod to Date or (S)elective Dates    : P

                       Starting Date    : 01/02/08
                       Ending Date      : 06/02/08

                 (S)elective Account Numbers or (A)ll      : A

                       Starting Account No.   : [B]
                       Ending Account No.     : [E]
                   ** ALIGN PRINTER TO TOP OF FORM **

                 Enter <PROCESS> or <EXIT>    : .




Ready                                                  NUM    ↑↓←→
```

Figure 7-4 Summary Current Period Report

```
06/02/08                    SUMMARY CURRENT PERIOD REPORT FOR 01/02/08 - 06/02/08              Page 1
                                        Student: Lois Fitzpatrick
                                             All Accounts
```

Acct No	Name	Phone No.	Bal Fwd	Charges	Receipts	Adjust	Balance
305	Viajo, Catherine A	(916) 694-3015		40.00			40.00
306	Cusack, Christine G	(916) 234-1795		98.00			98.00
307	Wyatt, John	(906) 795-2806		73.00			73.00
308	Frost, William	(916) 326-0531		71.00		71.00	0.00
309	Perez, Juan	(917) 836-4213		50.00			50.00
310	Stanch, Rebecca	(906) 826-9813		160.00			160.00
311	Vega, Roberto R	(906) 845-8126		200.00			200.00
315	Morgan, Margeret F	(907) 791-3325		126.00			126.00
316	Barker, Sharon	(916) 331-7604		89.00			89.00
317	Lopez, Sonia A	(917) 633-0219		55.00			55.00
318	Brinkman, Gary	(906) 729-4819		418.00			418.00
319	Miles, Wayne P	(906) 281-7305		123.00	123.00		0.00
320	Ramirez, Leanna M	(907) 431-0798		55.00	10.00		45.00
321	Marchese, Anna S	(916) 698-0102		40.00	40.00		0.00
322	Santos, Paul R	(917) 379-0834		147.00	16.00		131.00
323	Weiland, Candace	(917) 363-2963		88.00	88.00		0.00
324	Hatcher, Craig M	(917) 795-6115		73.00	61.35	11.65	0.00
325	Roberts, Ashleigh K	(907) 761-2315		93.00	84.68	8.32	0.00
326	Scheller, Denise L	(917) 741-1143		126.00	110.43		15.57
327	Fitzpatrick, Mark P	(906) 691-2538		243.00	223.36	19.64	0.00
328	Penny, Robert	(906) 976-2733		111.00	130.00		-19.00
329	Knifert, John	(906) 542-7893		71.00	8.00		63.00
330	Zapola, Karen L	(906) 472-8673		155.00	155.00		0.00
331	Jones, Elizabeth	(906) 893-2815		65.00	5.00		60.00
	TOTALS :		0.00	2770.00	1054.82	110.61	1604.57

```
                    **** A/R Reconciliation Not Performed - Unclosed Daily Items  ****


                ** Report Does Not Include Guarantors with ONLY Unapplied Credit Balances  **
```

NOTE: The reports will be based on the account activity entered to date. Therefore, the report information will vary by the unit exercises that have been completed.

EXERCISE 3: SYSTEM FINANCIAL SUMMARY REPORT

GOAL(S): In this exercise, you will generate a System Financial Summary Report.

1. Generate the System Financial Summary Report based on the following information:

   a. Select printer.

   b. Generate the report for all doctors.

   c. Show receipts and adjusts analysis.

   d. Do not skip financially inactive doctors.

   e. Answer Y for page on doctor.

   f. Compare your screen to Figure 7-5, System Financial Summary Report Selection Screen, and press F1 to print the report. Compare your printout to Figure 7-6.

Figure 7-5   System Financial Summary Report Selection Screen

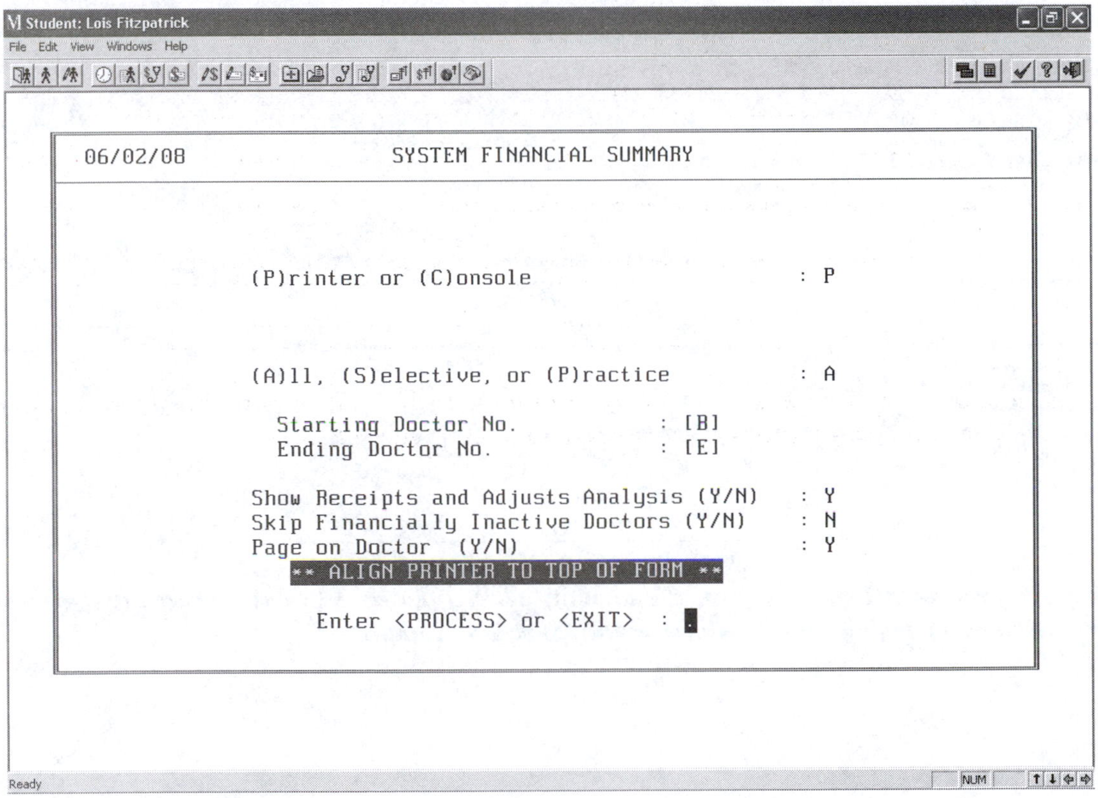

Figure 7-6a   System Financial Summary – James Monroe

```
06/02/08                        SYSTEM FINANCIAL SUMMARY - DETAIL                      Page 1
                                     James T Monroe MD (1)


--------------------------------------------------------------------------------------------
Dates                    Charges   Receipts   Adjustments   Net A/R   Total A/R   # Proc.  Col %
--------------------------------------------------------------------------------------------
01/02/08 - 02/16/08       407.00     18.00        0.00       389.00     389.00        7    4.4%
01/02/08 - 02/16/08       407.00     18.00        0.00       389.00     389.00        7    4.4%
--------------------------------------------------------------------------------------------


                           Receipts Analysis for : James T Monroe MD (1)
--------------------------------------------------------------------------------------------
             Net Receipts                PTD                YTD
--------------------------------------------------------------------------------------------
             Medicare                    0.00               0.00
             Insurance                   0.00               0.00
             Capitation Payments        60.00             180.00
             Patient                    18.00              18.00
             Other                       0.00               0.00
                                     ----------         ----------
             Total Receipts            78.00             198.00
             Refunds                     0.00               0.00
                                     ==========         ==========
             Gross Receipts            78.00             198.00


                           Adjustments for : James T Monroe MD (1)
--------------------------------------------------------------------------------------------
Adjustments          PTD         YTD       Adjustments              PTD         YTD
--------------------------------------------------------------------------------------------
1) General Adjustment   0.00     0.00      2) General Write-Off     0.00        0.00
3) Medicare Adjustment  0.00     0.00      4) Medicare Write-Off    0.00        0.00
5) HMO Adj & Write-Off  0.00     0.00
                     ==========  ==========
Total Adjustments       0.00     0.00


                            Refunds for : James T Monroe MD (1)
--------------------------------------------------------------------------------------------
Refunds              PTD         YTD       Refunds                  PTD         YTD
--------------------------------------------------------------------------------------------
0) Unspecified Refund   0.00     0.00      1) Incorrect Data Entry  0.00        0.00
2) Overpayment Refund   0.00     0.00      3) Returned Check        0.00        0.00
96) Acct Transfer To    0.00     0.00     97) Acct Transfer From    0.00        0.00
98) Cross-Alloc To      0.00     0.00     99) Cross-Alloc From      0.00        0.00
                     ==========  ==========
Total Refunds           0.00     0.00
```

NOTE: *The reports will be based on the account activity entered to date. Therefore, the report information will vary by the unit exercises that have been completed.*

Figure 7-6b   System Financial Summary – Frances Simpson

```
06/02/08                        SYSTEM FINANCIAL SUMMARY - DETAIL                    Page 2
                                  Frances D Simpson M.D. (2)


----------------------------------------------------------------------------------------------
Dates                  Charges    Receipts    Adjustments   Net A/R   Total A/R   # Proc.  Col %
----------------------------------------------------------------------------------------------
01/02/08 - 02/16/08     339.00     295.00        0.00        44.00      44.00         9    87.0%
01/02/08 - 02/16/08     339.00     295.00        0.00        44.00      44.00         9    87.0%
----------------------------------------------------------------------------------------------


                       Receipts Analysis for : Frances D Simpson M.D. (2)
----------------------------------------------------------------------------------------------
               Net Receipts                    PTD                 YTD
----------------------------------------------------------------------------------------------
               Medicare                        0.00                0.00
               Insurance                       0.00                0.00
               Capitation Payments             0.00                0.00
               Patient                       295.00              295.00
               Other                           0.00                0.00
                                          ----------          ----------
               Total Receipts                295.00              295.00
               Refunds                         0.00                0.00
                                          ==========          ==========
               Gross Receipts                295.00              295.00


                       Adjustments for : Frances D Simpson M.D. (2)
----------------------------------------------------------------------------------------------
Adjustments            PTD          YTD      Adjustments              PTD          YTD
----------------------------------------------------------------------------------------------
1) General Adjustment    0.00       0.00     2) General Write-Off      0.00        0.00
3) Medicare Adjustment   0.00       0.00     4) Medicare Write-Off     0.00        0.00
5) HMO Adj & Write-Off   0.00       0.00
                    ==========  ==========
Total Adjustments        0.00       0.00


                       Refunds for : Frances D Simpson M.D. (2)
----------------------------------------------------------------------------------------------
Refunds                PTD          YTD      Refunds                  PTD          YTD
----------------------------------------------------------------------------------------------
0) Unspecified Refund    0.00       0.00     1) Incorrect Data Entry   0.00        0.00
2) Overpayment Refund    0.00       0.00     3) Returned Check         0.00        0.00
96) Acct Transfer To     0.00       0.00     97) Acct Transfer From    0.00        0.00
98) Cross-Alloc To       0.00       0.00     99) Cross-Alloc From      0.00        0.00
                    ==========  ==========
Total Refunds            0.00       0.00
```

NOTE: *The reports will be based on the account activity entered to date. Therefore, the report information will vary by the unit exercises that have been completed.*

Figure 7-6c   System Financial Summary – Sydney Carrington

```
06/02/08                        SYSTEM FINANCIAL SUMMARY - DETAIL                         Page 3
                                   Sydney J Carrington M.D. (3)


-----------------------------------------------------------------------------------------------
Dates                         Charges    Receipts   Adjustments    Net A/R    Total A/R   # Proc.   Col %
-----------------------------------------------------------------------------------------------
01/02/08 - 02/16/08            191.00      20.00         0.00       171.00      171.00         6     10.5%
01/02/08 - 02/16/08            191.00      20.00         0.00       171.00      171.00         6     10.5%
-----------------------------------------------------------------------------------------------


                        Receipts Analysis for : Sydney J Carrington M.D. (3)
-----------------------------------------------------------------------------------------------
               Net Receipts                     PTD                  YTD
-----------------------------------------------------------------------------------------------
               Medicare                         0.00                 0.00
               Insurance                        0.00                 0.00
               Capitation Payments            235.00               625.00
               Patient                         20.00               437.00
               Other                            0.00                 0.00
                                          ----------           ----------
               Total Receipts                 255.00             1,062.00
               Refunds                          0.00                 0.00
                                          ==========           ==========
               Gross Receipts                 255.00             1,062.00


                        Adjustments for : Sydney J Carrington M.D. (3)
-----------------------------------------------------------------------------------------------
Adjustments            PTD          YTD      Adjustments              PTD          YTD
-----------------------------------------------------------------------------------------------
1) General Adjustment    0.00         0.00   2) General Write-Off       0.00         0.00
3) Medicare Adjustment   0.00         0.00   4) Medicare Write-Off      0.00         0.00
5) HMO Adj & Write-Off   0.00         0.00
                    ==========   ==========
Total Adjustments        0.00         0.00


                        Refunds for : Sydney J Carrington M.D. (3)
-----------------------------------------------------------------------------------------------
Refunds                PTD          YTD      Refunds                  PTD          YTD
-----------------------------------------------------------------------------------------------
0) Unspecified Refund    0.00         0.00   1) Incorrect Data Entry    0.00         0.00
2) Overpayment Refund    0.00         0.00   3) Returned Check          0.00         0.00
96) Acct Transfer To     0.00         0.00   97) Acct Transfer From     0.00         0.00
98) Cross-Alloc To       0.00         0.00   99) Cross-Alloc From       0.00         0.00
                    ==========   ==========
Total Refunds            0.00         0.00
```

NOTE: The reports will be based on the account activity entered to date. Therefore, the report information will vary by the unit exercises that have been completed.

Figure 7-6d System Financial Summary – Sandra Shiller

```
06/02/08                    SYSTEM FINANCIAL SUMMARY - DETAIL              Page 4
                                Sandra A Shiller, RPT (4)

--------------------------------------------------------------------------------
Dates                 Charges    Receipts   Adjustments   Net A/R   Total A/R   # Proc.   Col %
--------------------------------------------------------------------------------
01/02/08 - 02/16/08    0.00       0.00        0.00         0.00       0.00         0       0.0%
01/02/08 - 02/16/08    0.00       0.00        0.00         0.00       0.00         0       0.0%
--------------------------------------------------------------------------------


                    Receipts Analysis for : Sandra A Shiller, RPT (4)
--------------------------------------------------------------------------------
          Net Receipts                    PTD              YTD
--------------------------------------------------------------------------------
          Medicare                        0.00             0.00
          Insurance                       0.00             0.00
          Capitation Payments             0.00             0.00
          Patient                         0.00             0.00
          Other                           0.00             0.00
                                       ----------       ----------
          Total Receipts                  0.00             0.00
          Refunds                         0.00             0.00
                                       ==========       ==========
          Gross Receipts                  0.00             0.00


                    Adjustments for : Sandra A Shiller, RPT (4)
--------------------------------------------------------------------------------
Adjustments         PTD        YTD     Adjustments                 PTD        YTD
--------------------------------------------------------------------------------
1) General Adjustment   0.00    0.00   2) General Write-Off        0.00       0.00
3) Medicare Adjustment  0.00    0.00   4) Medicare Write-Off       0.00       0.00
5) HMO Adj & Write-Off  0.00    0.00
                    ==========  ==========
Total Adjustments       0.00    0.00


                    Refunds for : Sandra A Shiller, RPT (4)
--------------------------------------------------------------------------------
Refunds             PTD        YTD     Refunds                     PTD        YTD
--------------------------------------------------------------------------------
0) Unspecified Refund   0.00    0.00   1) Incorrect Data Entry     0.00       0.00
2) Overpayment Refund   0.00    0.00   3) Returned Check           0.00       0.00
96) Acct Transfer To    0.00    0.00   97) Acct Transfer From      0.00       0.00
98) Cross-Alloc To      0.00    0.00   99) Cross-Alloc From        0.00       0.00
                    ==========  ==========
Total Refunds           0.00    0.00
```

NOTE: *The reports will be based on the account activity entered to date. Therefore, the report information will vary by the unit exercises that have been completed.*

Figure 7-6e   System Financial Summary – Totals for Practice

```
06/02/08                        SYSTEM FINANCIAL SUMMARY                        Page 5
                                  TOTALS FOR PRACTICE
                      PERIOD-TO-DATE TOTALS FOR 01/02/08 - 02/16/08


------------------------------------------------------------------------------------------
Doctor                  Charges   Receipts  Adjustments   Net A/R   Total A/R   # Proc.  Col %
------------------------------------------------------------------------------------------
1. James T Monroe MD     407.00     18.00       0.00      389.00     389.00        7     4.4%
2. Frances D Simpson M.D. 339.00    295.00      0.00       44.00      44.00        9    87.0%
3. Sydney J Carrington M.D. 191.00   20.00      0.00      171.00     171.00        6    10.5%
4. Sandra A Shiller, RPT   0.00      0.00       0.00        0.00       0.00        0     0.0%
------------------------------------------------------------------------------------------
TOTALS                   937.00    333.00       0.00      604.00     604.00       22    35.5%
Practice Totals :        937.00    333.00       0.00      604.00     604.00       22    35.5%


                      YEAR-TO-DATE TOTALS FOR 01/02/08 - 02/16/08

------------------------------------------------------------------------------------------
Doctor                  Charges   Receipts  Adjustments   Net A/R   Total A/R   # Proc.  Col %
------------------------------------------------------------------------------------------
1. James T Monroe MD     407.00     18.00       0.00      389.00     389.00        7     4.4%
2. Frances D Simpson M.D. 339.00    295.00      0.00       44.00      44.00        9    87.0%
3. Sydney J Carrington M.D. 191.00   20.00      0.00      171.00     171.00        6    10.5%
4. Sandra A Shiller, RPT   0.00      0.00       0.00        0.00       0.00        0     0.0%
------------------------------------------------------------------------------------------
TOTALS :                 937.00    333.00       0.00      604.00     604.00       22    35.5%
Practice Totals :        937.00    333.00       0.00      604.00     604.00       22    35.5%


                            Receipts Analysis for Practice
------------------------------------------------------------------------------------------
              Net Receipts                 PTD                 YTD
------------------------------------------------------------------------------------------
              Medicare                     0.00                0.00
              Insurance                    0.00                0.00
              Capitation Payments        295.00              805.00
              Patient                    333.00              750.00
              Other                        0.00                0.00
                                      ----------          ----------
              Total Receipts             628.00            1,555.00
              Refunds                      0.00                0.00
                                      ==========          ==========
              Gross Receipts             628.00            1,555.00
```

NOTE: The reports will be based on the account activity entered to date. Therefore, the report information will vary by the unit exercises that have been completed.

Figure 7-6f System Financial Summary – Adjustments for Practice

```
06/02/08                          SYSTEM FINANCIAL SUMMARY                      Page 6
                                    Adjustments for Practice


--------------------------------------------------------------------------------------
Adjustments              PTD           YTD    Adjustments              PTD           YTD
--------------------------------------------------------------------------------------
 1) General Adjustment    0.00          0.00   2) General Write-Off     0.00          0.00
 3) Medicare Adjustment   0.00          0.00   4) Medicare Write-Off    0.00          0.00
 5) HMO Adj & Write-Off   0.00          0.00
                      ==========    ==========
Total Adjustments         0.00          0.00


--------------------------------------------------------------------------------------
Refunds                  PTD           YTD    Refunds                  PTD           YTD
--------------------------------------------------------------------------------------
 0) Unspecified Refund    0.00          0.00   1) Incorrect Data Entry  0.00          0.00
 2) Overpayment Refund    0.00          0.00   3) Returned Check        0.00          0.00
96) Acct Transfer To      0.00          0.00  97) Acct Transfer From    0.00          0.00
98) Cross-Alloc To        0.00          0.00  99) Cross-Alloc From      0.00          0.00
                      ==========    ==========
Total Refunds             0.00          0.00
```

NOTE: The reports will be based on the account activity entered to date. Therefore, the report information will vary by the unit exercises that have been completed.

EXERCISE 4: PRINTING PATIENT STATEMENTS

GOAL(S): In this exercise, you will print patient statements.

1. Print patient statements based on the following information:

   a. Do not run a trial.

   b. Accept the default date.

   c. Choose the statements to be printed for all accounts in account order.

   d. Print the patient statements (Figures 7-7 and 7-8).

NOTE: You will generate 23 patient statements similar to Figure 7-8. Your statement for Mark Fitzpatrick may vary depending on which exercises you have completed in previous units.

Figure 7-7 Patient Statement Selection Screen

```
06/02/08                PATIENT STATEMENTS ROUTINE

  Trial (Y/N) : N   Finance Charge (Y/N) : N   Cycle (Y/N/Restart)  : N

  Enter Bill-Thru-Date or <CR> for  06/02/08              : 06/02/08

  Order : (A)ccount #, (N)ame, (D)octor or (Z)ip          : A
  Scope : (A)ll, (S)elective, (R)ange, (B)ill Type, or (D)elinquent : A

                      Patient  1 : ......
                      Patient  2 : ......
                      Patient  3 : ......
                      Patient  4 : ......
                      Patient  5 : ......
                      Patient  6 : ......
                      Patient  7 : ......
                      Patient  8 : ......
                      Patient  9 : ......
                      Patient 10 : ......

                 Enter <PROCESS> or <EXIT>          : █
```

Figure 7-8 Sample Patient Statement – Mark Fitzpatrick

```
                        Student: Lois Fitzpatrick
                        34 Sycamore St. Suite 300
                        Madison Ca. 95653
                           (916) 398-7654



          Mark P Fitzpatrick              327           06/02/08
          1735 Parker Street
          Apt. 5A                                       Page No. 1
          Los Angeles CA 98706


   Date         Description of Transaction          Amount         Ins
   ----------------------------------------------------------------------
                Balance Forward                       .00
   02/02/08     Office Estb: Comprhn                 85.00          *
   02/02/08     Urinalysis by dip st                  8.00          *
   02/02/08     X-Ray Spine. Cerv 4                 150.00          *
   01/11/08     Payment .... Thank Y                 -2.00
   06/02/08     Payment - Pan Americ               -221.36
   06/02/08     General Write-Off                    -6.66
   06/02/08     General Write-Off                    -1.77
   06/02/08     General Write-Off                   -11.21
   ----------------------------------------------------------------------


                                                      .00

                    *Insurance Pending:               .00

                    Total Due From Patient:           .00

   Next Appointment :

   Aging:      CURRENT      31 - 60      61 - 90      91 - 120     121 - up

                 .00          .00          .00          .00          .00

              ** Statement Due Upon Receipt * Thank You **
```

U N I T   8

Advanced Functions

In the unit exercises that follow, you will refund an overpayment, remove credit for a bad check, use Auto Pay from the insurance, rebill an insurance claim, and add a patient to a hospital rounds report. In addition, you will print an aging report and print patient data.

EXERCISE 1: REFUNDING AN OVERPAYMENT

ROBERT PENNY; ACCOUNT 328

GOAL(S): In this exercise, you will correct a mistake made by the medical office during the posting procedure by refunding an overpayment.

Robert Penny was seen on 02/16/2008 for an office visit with lab work. He wrote a check for the charges totaling $111. The payment was mistakenly entered as $130. The money was applied to his visit leaving a $19 unapplied credit. The account needs to be updated with a refund from the unapplied credit.

1. Based on the information above, retrieve Robert Penny's account at the Payment Entry screen and complete a refund of $19. Enter the refund as an incorrect data entry. Compare your screens to Figures 8-1 and 8-2.

Figure 8-1   Selecting Unapplied Credit

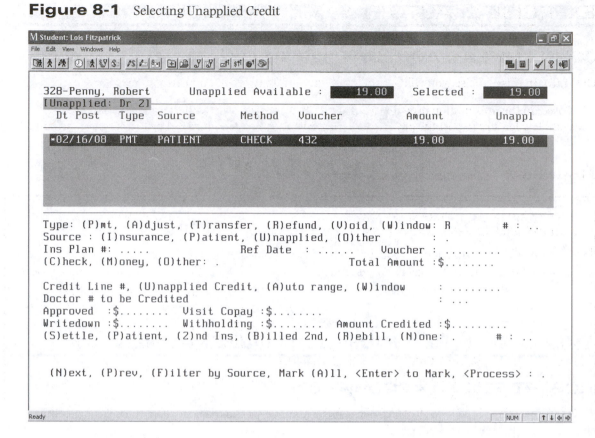

Figure 8-2   Posting a Refund

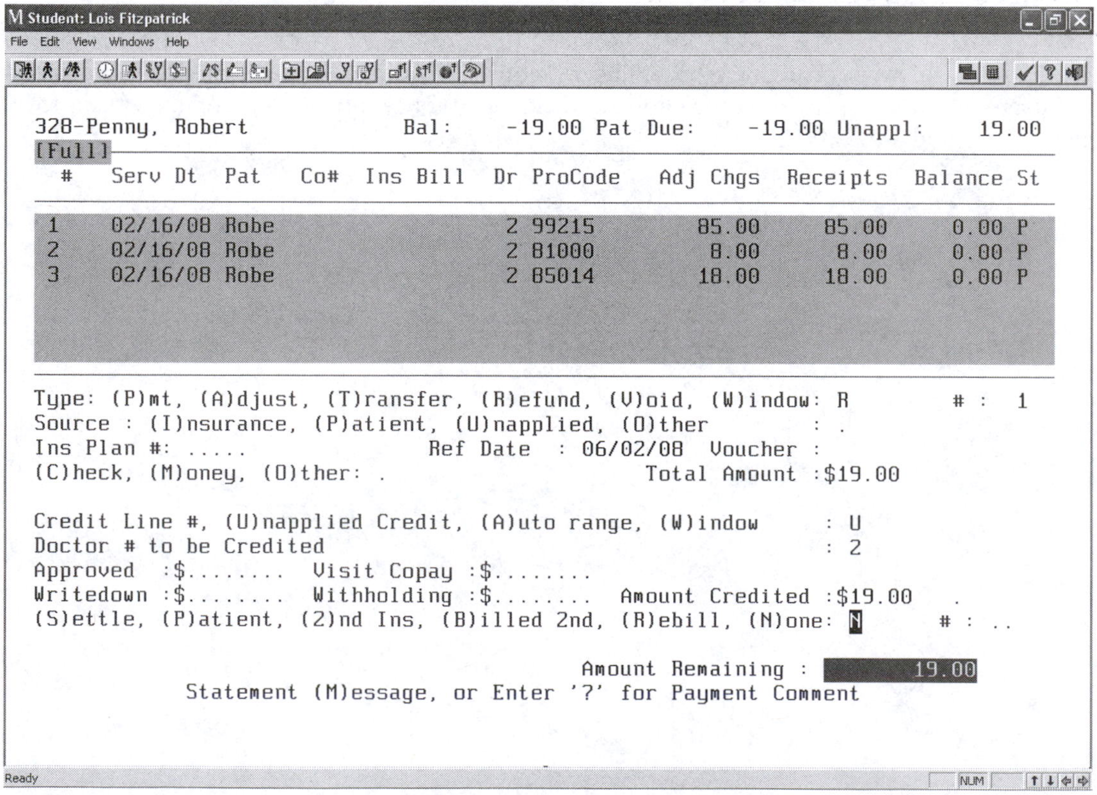

EXERCISE 2: AUTO PAY WITH AN INSURANCE CHECK

JOHN KNIFERT; ACCOUNT 329

GOAL(S): In this exercise, you will use the Auto Pay feature to credit an insurance check.

1. Based on the information provided from Figure 8-3, retrieve John Knifert's account and use the Auto Pay feature to post the payment. Compare your screen to Figure 8-4 before pressing the F1 key.

Figure 8-3 Pan American Check – Knifert

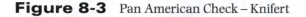

```
PAN AMERICAN LIFE INSURANCE COMPANY                          623103
GROUP INSURANCE OPERATIONS  LOS ANGELES, CALIFORNIA


                                        CONTROLLER NUMBER  9087654839

                                        POLICYHOLDER NAME    WOODSIDE FD
                                        INSURED NAME         JOHN KNIFERT
                                        CLAIMANT NAME        JOHN KNIFERT
                                        DATE(S) OF SERVICE   02/16/08
PAY            SYDNEY CARRINGTON & ASSOCIATES
TO THE         34 SYCAMORE STREET
ORDER          SUITE 300                     MO. DAY YR        PAY
OF             MADISON, CALIFORNIA 95653     04 – 16 - 08      63.00

AMERICAN BANK                                   BY  M.K.Cist
Madison, California

⑈414012 000042⑊ 190151194611⑈
```

Figure 8-4 Payment Screen Before Posting

```
M Student: Lois Fitzpatrick                                                      _ □ X
File  Edit  View  Windows  Help
[toolbar icons]                                                          ▢ ▣ ✓ ? ⬌

   329-Knifert, John           Bal:      63.00 Pat Due:      0.00 Unappl:     0.00
   [Full]
    #   Serv Dt  Pat   Co#  Ins Bill   Dr ProCode   Adj Chgs  Receipts  Balance St

    1   02/16/08 John     7 02/16/08    1 99213        40.00      8.00    32.00 I
    2   02/16/08 John     7 02/16/08    1 87070        31.00      0.00    31.00 I




   Type: (P)mt, (A)djust, (T)ransfer, (R)efund, (V)oid, (W)indow: P        # : ..
   Source : (I)nsurance, (P)atient, (U)napplied, (O)ther      : I
   Ins Plan #:      7              Ref Date  : 06/02/08  Voucher : 623103
   (C)heck, (M)oney, (O)ther: C                 Total Amount :$63.00

   Credit Line #, (U)napplied Credit, (A)uto range, (W)indow    : A1-2
   Doctor # to be Credited                                      : ...
   Approved  :$........  Visit Copay :$........
   Writedown :$........  Withholding :$........  Amount Credited :$........
   (S)ettle, (P)atient, (2)nd Ins, (B)illed 2nd, (R)ebill, (N)one: N       # : ..
                            AUTOPAY
                                    Amount Remaining :           63.00
            Statement (M)essage, or Enter '?' for Payment Comment


Ready                                                              NUM    ↑↓⬌⬍
```

EXERCISE 3: REMOVING A BAD CHECK

KAREN ZAPOLA; ACCOUNT 330

GOAL(S): In this exercise, you will remove the credit for a bad check.

The bank has returned Karen Zapola's $155 check due to nonsufficient funds (see Figure 8-5).

1. Post a negative payment to Karen Zapola's account to restore the item balance to unpaid. Compare your screen to Figure 8-6, then press F1.

2. Post a refund to remove the credit from the doctor's receipts. Compare your screen to Figure 8-7, then press F1.

Figure 8-5 Returned Check

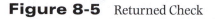

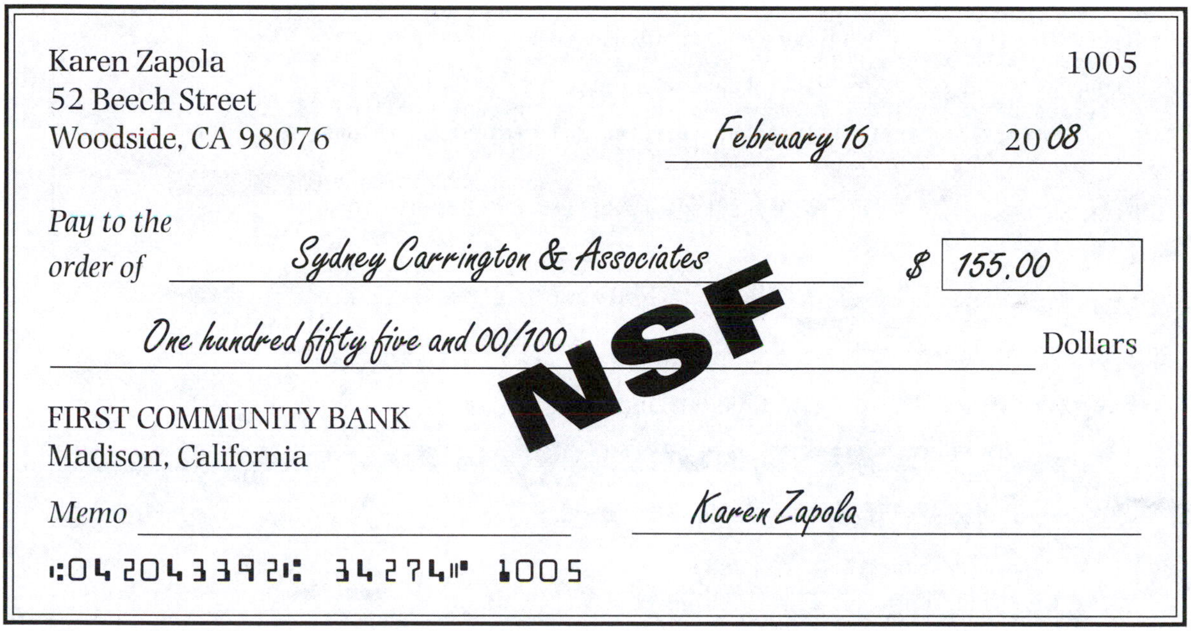

Karen Zapola   1005
52 Beech Street
Woodside, CA 98076   *February 16*   20 *08*

Pay to the
order of   *Sydney Carrington & Associates* $ 155.00

          One hundred fifty five and 00/100   NSF   Dollars

FIRST COMMUNITY BANK
Madison, California

Memo _____   *Karen Zapola*

⑆04 2043392⑆ 34274⑈ 1005

Figure 8-6   Payment Screen Before Posting Reversal

```
M Student: Lois Fitzpatrick                                                    _ [] X
File  Edit  View  Windows  Help

330-Zapola, Karen L          Bal:      0.00 Pat Due:      0.00 Unappl:      0.00
[Full]
   #   Serv Dt  Pat    Co#  Ins Bill  Dr ProCode    Adj Chgs   Receipts  Balance St

   1   02/16/08 Kare              2 99213        40.00     40.00     0.00 P
   2   02/16/08 Kare              2 71020        58.00     58.00     0.00 P
   3   02/16/08 Kare              2 93000        57.00     57.00     0.00 P


Type: (P)mt, (A)djust, (T)ransfer, (R)efund, (V)oid, (W)indow: P         # : ..
Source : (I)nsurance, (P)atient, (U)nappled, (O)ther       : P
Ins Plan #: ....           Ref Date  : 06/02/08  Voucher : 1005
(C)heck, (M)oney, (O)ther: C                Total Amount :$-155.00

Credit Line #, (U)nappled Credit, (A)uto range, (W)indow    : A1-3
Doctor # to be Credited                                     : ...
Approved  :$........  Visit Copay :$........
Writedown :$........  Withholding :$........  Amount Credited :$........
(S)ettle, (P)atient, (2)nd Ins, (B)illed 2nd, (R)ebill, (N)one: P      # : ..

                                  Amount Remaining :      -155.00
                     Transfer Responsibility to Patient                  .

Ready                                                           NUM    ↑↓←→
```

Figure 8-7   Removing the Credit Balance

```
M Student: Lois Fitzpatrick                                                    _ [] X
File  Edit  View  Windows  Help

330-Zapola, Karen L          Bal:      0.00 Pat Due:      0.00 Unappl:    155.00
[Full]
   #   Serv Dt  Pat    Co#  Ins Bill  Dr ProCode    Adj Chgs   Receipts  Balance St

   1   02/16/08 Kare              2 99213        40.00      0.00    40.00 P
   2   02/16/08 Kare              2 71020        58.00      0.00    58.00 P
   3   02/16/08 Kare              2 93000        57.00      0.00    57.00 P


Type: (P)mt, (A)djust, (T)ransfer, (R)efund, (V)oid, (W)indow: R         # :  3
Source : (I)nsurance, (P)atient, (U)nappled, (O)ther       : .
Ins Plan #: .....          Ref Date  : 06/02/08  Voucher :
(C)heck, (M)oney, (O)ther: .                Total Amount :$155.00

Credit Line #, (U)nappled Credit, (A)uto range, (W)indow    : U
Doctor # to be Credited                                     : 2
Approved  :$........  Visit Copay :$........
Writedown :$........  Withholding :$........  Amount Credited :$155.00   .
(S)ettle, (P)atient, (2)nd Ins, (B)illed 2nd, (R)ebill, (N)one: N      # : ..

                                  Amount Remaining :      155.00
          Statement (M)essage, or Enter '?' for Payment Comment

Ready                                                           NUM    ↑↓←→
```

EXERCISE 4: REBILLING A LOST CLAIM

ELIZABETH JONES; ACCOUNT 331

GOAL(S): In this exercise, you will rebill a lost insurance claim.

The insurance plan, Epsilon Life & Casualty, has no record of ever receiving a claim on Elizabeth Jones for her 02/16/2008 visit. You must rebill the claim using an adjustment of zero dollars.

1. Using the information provided, retrieve Elizabeth Jones' account and rebill the claim that has been lost. Be sure to complete the rebill for each procedure. When you have rebilled each item, compare your screen to Figure 8-8.

Figure 8-8   After Rebill of Item – Jones

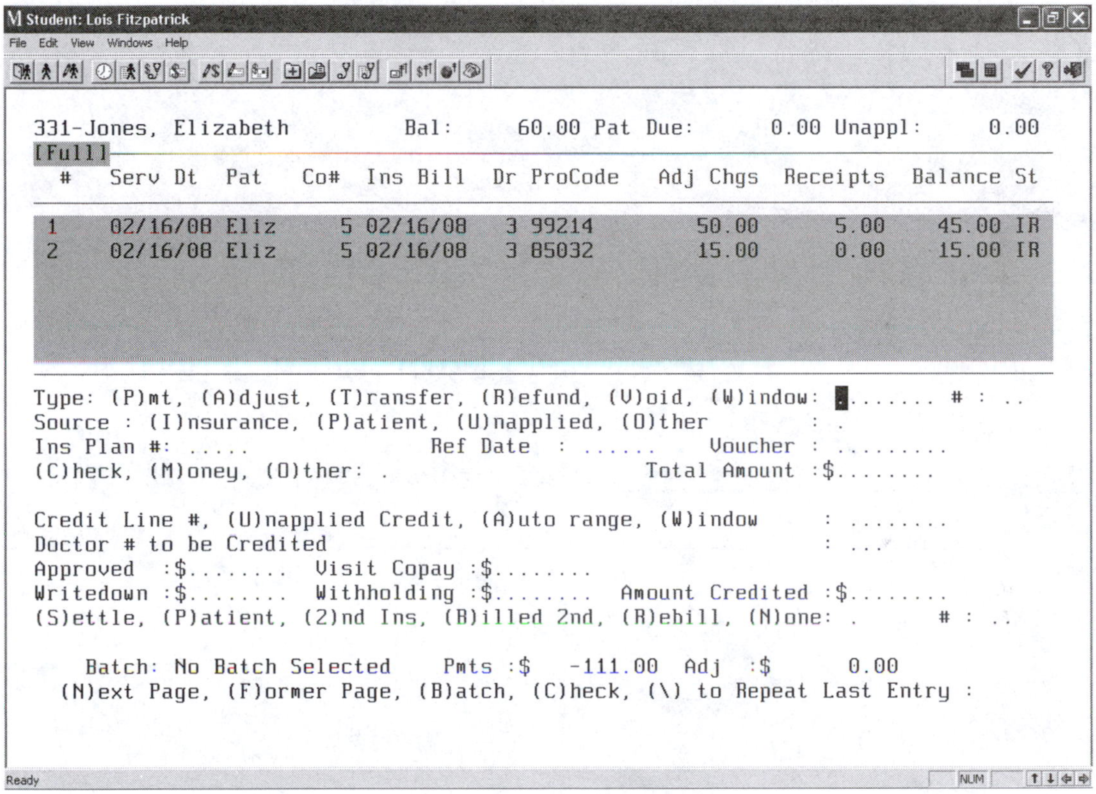

EXERCISE 5: HOSPITAL ROUNDS

ROSS WALKER; ACCOUNT 332

GOAL(S): In this exercise, you will add a patient to a hospital rounds report.

Ross Walker has been complaining of intense migraine headaches. Previous treatments have not resolved the condition. Dr. Carrington wants to admit Ross Walker to Madison General Hospital for two days and schedule an MRI and CAT scan.

1. Based on the information provided, add Ross Walker to Dr. Carrington's hospital rounds report.

   a. Have the entry appear on Dr. Carrington's rounds report. Accept the default referring doctor.

   b. Leave Room No. and Hospital Pat # blank.

2. Ross will be admitted today (06/02/2008).

3. Ross' admission to the hospital is elective.

4. Compare your screen to Figure 8-9.

Figure 8-9   Hospital Rounds

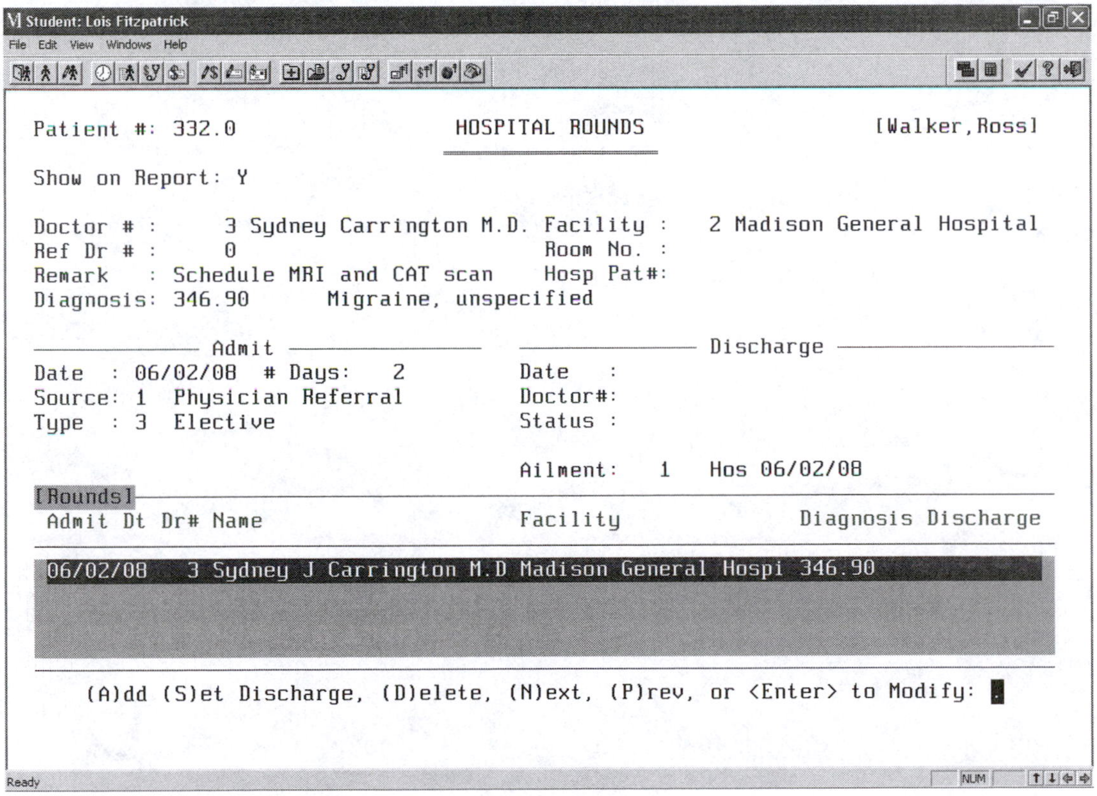

EXERCISE 6: RUNNING AGING REPORT

GOAL(S): In this exercise, you will print an Aging Analysis by Practice report.

You are asked to run an aging report that compares patient and insurance due portions of accounts.

1. Print an Aging Report, selecting (A)nalysis level for the medical practice.

2. Accept the default responses for All Procedure Locations. Compare your screen to Figure 8-10.

NOTE: Your Aging Report may vary from Figure 8-11 depending on exercises from previous units.

Figure 8-10   Aging Report Selection Screen

```
06/02/08                          AGING REPORT

    (D)etail, (S)ummary, or (A)nalysis                 : A
    (A)ccount, (P)at., (I)ns.#, (C)arrier or (D)octor  : D


(A)ll, (S)elective, (P)ractice                         : P
    Starting No.     : [B]
    Ending No.       : [E]

Starting Age Cat. (1-6, S) : 1   Ending Age Cat. (1-6) : 6
    Cat 1  Range: [B] to   30    Cat 4  Range:  91 to 120
    Cat 2  Range:  31 to   60    Cat 5  Range: 121 to 150
    Cat 3  Range:  61 to   90    Cat 6  Range: 151 to [E]

(A)ll or (S)elective Procedure Location                : A

Skip if Pmt Since                                      : 06/02/08
Include Status (A)ll,  (R)ange, (S)elective : A
Exclude Status (N)one, (R)ange, (S)elective : N
            Enter <PROCESS> or <EXIT> : 
```

** ALIGN PRINTER TO TOP OF FORM **

Figure 8-11 System Aging Analysis

```
06/02/08                    SYSTEM AGING ANALYSIS BY DOCTOR                    Page 1
                               Student: Lois Fitzpatrick
                               SUMMARY FOR PRACTICE
                               All Procedure Locations

     -------------------------------------------------------------------------------
                      0 - 30      31 - 60     61 - 90     91 - 120    121 - 150    151 +
     -------------------------------------------------------------------------------
     Patient  :       205.00       0.00        0.00         0.00        0.00       0.00
        %     :       100.0        0.0%        0.0%         0.0%        0.0%       0.0%
     Insurance :     1450.57       0.00        0.00        60.00        0.00       0.00
        %     :        96.0%       0.0%        0.0%         4.0%        0.0%       0.0%
     -------------------------------------------------------------------------------
     Totals   :      1655.57       0.00        0.00        60.00        0.00       0.00
        %     :        96.5%       0.0%        0.0%         3.5%        0.0%       0.0%
     -------------------------------------------------------------------------------


     Total Patient Receivables    :       205.00       11.9%      (Date-Patient-Responsible)
     Total Insurance Receivables  :      1510.57       88.1%      (Date-Company-Billed)
     Total Open Items             :      1715.57      100.0%      (Summation-of-Above)


              **** A/R Reconciliation Not Performed - Unclosed Daily Items ****

                 **** Report Totals Do NOT Reflect Unapplied Credits ****
```

EXERCISE 7: PRINTING PATIENT DATA

GOAL(S): In this exercise, you will print the Insurance Plan and Insured Party Information from the Display Patient Data screen.

Since Ross Walker is being admitted to the hospital, you want to be familiar with his insurance coverage.

1. From the Display Patient Data screen, print the hardcopies of Ross Walker's insurance coverage.

2. Since he has dual coverage, be sure to position the light bar on each plan before selecting (H)ard copy. Compare your reports to Figures 8-12 and 8-13.

Figure 8-12 Guarantor Insurance Coverage

```
   Patient #: 332.0          GUARANTOR INSURANCE COVERAGE        [Walker, Ross]

                          ==================================

   Policyholder: Jacqueline Walker             SSN     : 281-65-3243
   Carrier : EPSLON        Epsilon Life & Casualty   Policy # : 281653243
   Plan #  : 5             Epsilon Life & Casualty   Commercial Ins Co Plan
   Dates-From:             To:


   Attn  :                                     Deductible  : 300.00
   Phone : (800) 908-7654                       Visit Copay :   0.00
   Fax   :                              Group  :
   Elig  :                                       Randall, Inc.
   Auth  :                              Insured: Jacqueline Walker
                                        User Note :



   -----------------------------------------------------------------------
   Plan#      Plan Name              Effective Dates     Assign      Note
   -----------------------------------------------------------------------
    5.1       Epsilon Life & Casualty        -              YY
    7.0       Pan American Health Ins.       -              YY
   -----------------------------------------------------------------------
```

Figure 8-13 Account Insurance Coverage

```
Patient #: 332.0          GUARANTOR INSURANCE COVERAGE        [Walker, Ross]

                          ===================================

Policyholder: Ross M Walker                  SSN     : 794-85-5882
Carrier : PANAMC      Pan Amercian Health Ins.  Policy # : RP259867
Plan #  : 7           Pan Amercian Health Ins.  Commercial Ins Co Plan
Dates-From:                    To:

Attn  :                                      Deductible  : 0.00
Phone : (213) 456-7654                       Visit Copay : 0.00
Fax   :                          Group :  IBM
Elig  :                                      Group Unnamed
Auth  :                          Insured: Ross M Walker
                                 User Note :


---------------------------------------------------------------------------
Plan#      Plan Name                Effective Dates     Assign      Note
---------------------------------------------------------------------------
 5.1       Epsilon Life & Casualty       -               YY
 7.0       Pan American Health Ins.      -               YY
---------------------------------------------------------------------------
```

EXERCISE 8: OPEN ITEMS

GOAL(S): In this exercise, you will print Open Items from the Display Patient Data screen.

Since Karen Zapola's check bounced from her 02/16/2008 visit, you want to print the account open items to show the detail of the credit back to the account.

1. Retrieve Karen Zapola's account at the Display Patient Data screen.

2. From Open Items, print a hard copy of each procedure on 02/16/2008 showing that the check was applied and then the charges were credited back to the account.

3. Give the reports to your instructor.

EXERCISE 9: INFORMATION ON ALL CHARGES AND PAYMENTS POSTED

GOAL(S): In this exercise, you will print the Financial History from the Display Patient Data screen.

1. Retrieve John Knifert's account from the Display Patient Data screen.

2. Print a hard copy of John Knifert's financial history showing the information on all charges and payments posted.

3. Give the report to your instructor.

U N I T 9

Today's Medical Office

In the unit exercises that follow, you will print a Patient Consent report, prepare an Authorization form, and record a disclosure on a patient's account.

NOTE: *The patients listed in Figure 9-1 may vary depending on exercises from previous units.*

EXERCISE 1: RUN THE PRIVACY SYSTEM PATIENT CONSENT REPORT

GOAL(S): In this exercise, you will print the Privacy System Patient Consent report.

1. Run the Privacy System Patient Consent report in account order for all accounts. Do not include comments.

2. Leave the "Only Patients Seen Since" field blank.

3. Print the report.

Figure 9-1a Patient Consent Report

```
06/02/08                    PATIENT CONSENT REPORT                    Page 1
                           Student: Lois Fitzpatrick
                            Account Order, All Dates
                         Comments Not Included, All Status

Patient #        Name                      DOL Visit            Status
---------------------------------------------------------------------------
   300.1      Walters Theresa L                                   Yes
   301.1      Carlos Helena                                       Yes
   302.0      Glenmore Edward R                                   Yes
   303.1      Monaco Nancy                                        Yes
   304.0      Monti Vincent A                                     Yes
   305.0      Viajo Catherine A            06/02/2008             Yes
   305.1      Viajo Michael                                       Yes
   306.0      Cusack Christine G           06/02/2008             Yes
   306.1      Cusack Richard                                      Yes
   307.0      Wyatt John                   06/02/2008             Yes
   308.0      Frost William                06/02/2008             Yes
   308.1      Frost Linda                  06/02/2008             Yes
   309.0      Perez juan                   06/02/2008             Yes
   310.0      Stanch Rebecca               06/02/2008             Yes
   310.1      Noonan Mathew                06/02/2008             Yes
   311.0      Vega Roberto R               06/02/2008             Yes
   312.0      Salvani William                                     Yes
   312.1      Salvani Christoper                                  Yes
   312.2      Salvani Kyle M                                      Yes
   313.0      Stein Erin R                                        Yes
   314.0      Fuentas Carmen P                                    Yes
   314.1      Fuentas David                                       Yes
   315.0      Morgan Margaret F            01/10/2008             Yes
   315.1      Morgan Brian                                        Yes
   315.2      Morgan Peter                                        Yes
   316.0      Barker Sharon                01/10/2008             Yes
   316.1      Barker Richard                                      Yes
   316.2      Barker Sarah                                        Yes
   317.0      Lopez Sonia A                06/02/2008             Yes
   318.0      Brinkman Gary                06/02/2008             Yes
   319.0      Miles Wayne P                06/02/2008             Yes
   319.1      Miles Sheila                                        Yes
   320.0      Ramirez Leanna M             06/02/2008             Yes
   321.0      Marchese Anna S              06/02/2008             Yes
   321.1      Marchese Nicholas                                   Yes
   322.0      Santos Paul R                06/02/2008             Yes
   322.1      Santos Carol                 06/02/2008             Yes
   323.0      Weiland Candace              06/02/2008             Yes
   323.1      Weiland Stephen              06/02/2008             Yes
   324.0      Hatcher Craig M              01/10/2008             Yes
   325.0      Roberts Ashleigh K           01/10/2008             Yes
   325.1      Roberts Renee                                       Yes
   326.0      Scheller Denise L            02/01/2003             Yes
   327.0      Fitzpatrick Mark P           02/01/2003             Yes
   327.1      Fitzpatrick Roberta                                 Yes
   328.0      Penny Robert                 02/15/2003             Yes
   329.0      Knifert John                 02/15/2003             Yes
   330.0      Zapola Karen L               02/15/2003             Yes
   331.0      Jones Elizabeth              02/15/2003             Yes
   332.0      Walker Ross M                                       Yes
   332.1      Walker Jacqueline                                   Yes
   333.0      Swindel Alan P                                      Yes
   333.1      Swindel Margaret                                    Yes
   333.2      Swindel Daniel                                      No
```

Figure 9-1b Patient Consent Report (continued)

```
06/02/08                    PATIENT CONSENT REPORT                      Page 2
                          Student: Lois Fitzpatrick
                          Account Order, All Dates
                        Comments Not Included, All Status


Patient #          Name                         DOL Visit            Status
------------------------------------------------------------------------------
   334.0      Berntson Allison                                         Yes
   335.0      Cantorelli Brittany R                                    Yes
   335.1      Rutger Donna                                             No
   336.0      Valentine Michael M                                      Yes


                              Total Yes       :    56
                              Total Limited   :     0
                              Total No        :     2
                              Total Revoked   :     0
                              Total Unknown   :     0
```

EXERCISE 2: PREPARE AN AUTHORIZATION FORM FOR A PATIENT

GOAL(S): In this exercise you will print an Authorization form for Daniel Swindel's wrestling coach.

Daniel Swindel needs an authorization form to be completed for his wrestling coach. In order to join the wrestling team, a sports physical is required for all students. Based on the following information, prepare an Authorization form for Daniel Swindel.

1. Retrieve Daniel Swindel's account from the Patient Privacy Records screen.

2. The form will be signed by Daniel's mother.

3. The Purpose of Disclosure is a sports physical.

4. Leave Contact Party blank and complete the following fields:

   a. Authorized Party: Fairview Middle School

   b. Attention: Wrestling Coach

   c. Address: 420 Hunter Avenue

   d. City: Madison

   e. State: CA

   f. Zip Code: 95653

5. The information to be disclosed are the results of the sports physical.

6. Compare your screen to Figure 9-2. Print the form. Compare your form to Figure 9-3.

Figure 9-2 Patient Privacy Authorization

Figure 9-3 Authorization to Disclose Patient Records

```
           AUTHORIZATION TO DISCLOSE PATIENT RECORDS


I hereby authorize Sydney Carrington & Associates P.A. to disclose individually
identifiable protected health information concerning the patient:

Daniel  Swindel
14 Bonekak Lane
Sacramento CA 94056

To:  Wrestling Coach
     420 Hunter Avenue
     Madison, CA 95653

For the purpose of:
Sports Physical


Information to be Disclosed:
Results of the sports physical


This Authorization is to remain in effect from  06/02/2008

I understand that I have the right to revoke this authorization  by notifying
the practice in writing until such time as a disclosure has been made based on
this authorization. In addition, I understand that my signing this
authorization is not required for the practice to provide me with health care
service, except if the sole purpose of the service is for the practice to
provide health care information to the authorized party named in this document.
Finally, I understand that the information disclosed pursuant to this
authorization may be redisclosed by the authorized party and no longer be
protected by the laws under which this authorization was created.




Signed _____     Date _____

Relation to Patient:  Parent
```

EXERCISE 3: RECORD A DISCLOSURE FOR A PATIENT

GOAL(S): In this exercise, you will record a disclosure for Daniel Swindel.

The results from Daniel's sports physical have been received. Based on the following information, prepare a record of disclosure, indicating that you have sent the results to his wrestling coach.

1. Retrieve Daniel Swindel's account from the Patient Privacy Records screen.

2. Select the sports physical and choose (D)isclosures.

3. Add a new disclosure record using the following information:

    a. Accept the default date for date of disclosure.

    b. Accept the default to disclose to the Authorized Party.

    c. Accept the default for the sports physical information to be disclosed.

4. Process the information. Compare your screen to Figure 9-4.

Figure 9-4 Disclosure Record

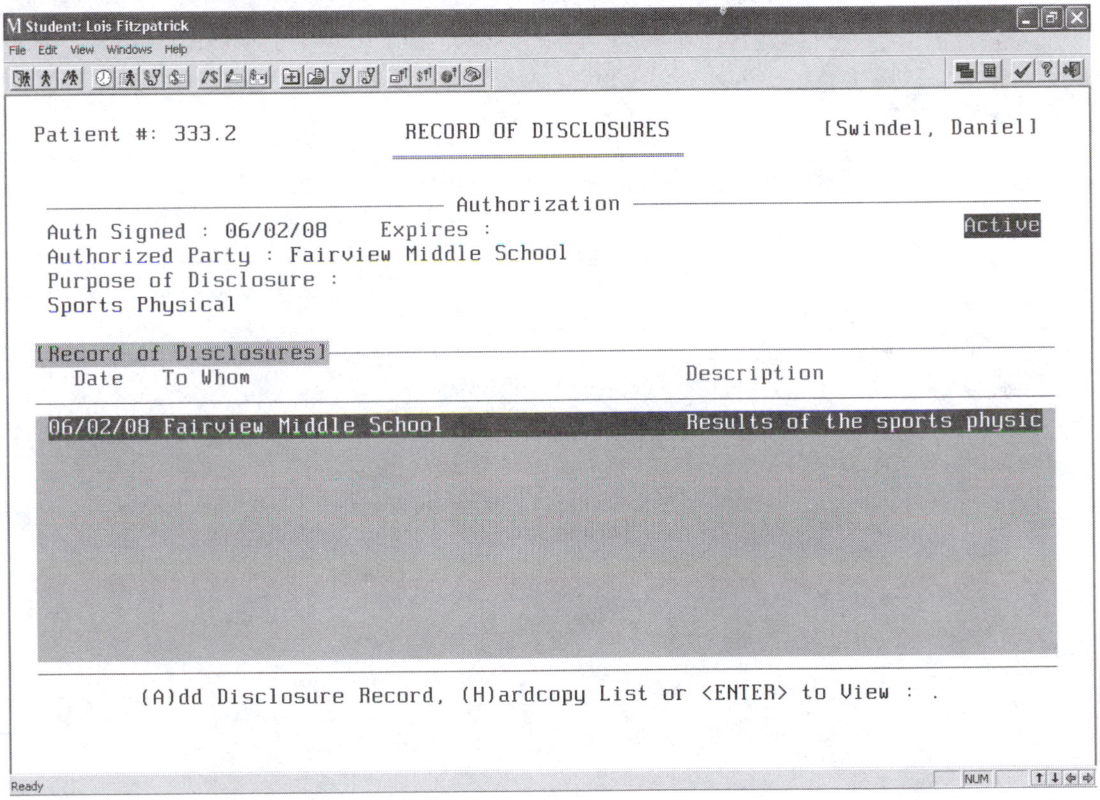

U N I T 10

Comprehensive Evaluation

The exercises that follow are intended to evaluate your understanding of The Medical Manager software. Complete each exercise in order, using the instructions and figures provided.

EXERCISE 1: ADD ACCOUNTS

1. Use Figures 10-1 through 10-5 to enter new patient accounts.

Figure 10-1   Patient Registration – Pamela Jermone

Patient Registration Form

Sydney Carrington & Associates
34 Sycamore Street ● Madison, CA 95653

FOR OFFICE USE ONLY	
ACCOUNT NO.:	337
DOCTOR:	#1
BILL TYPE:	11
EXTENDED INFO.:	2

TODAY'S DATE: _06/02/2008_

PATIENT INFORMATION

Jermone	Pamela	R.		Health Lab Corp.			
PATIENT LAST NAME	FIRST NAME	MI	SUFFIX	EMPLOYER OR SCHOOL NAME			
				5 Escada Road	Madison	CA	95653
MAILING ADDRESS	CITY	STATE	ZIP CODE	EMPLOYER OR SCHOOL ADDRESS	CITY	STATE	ZIP CODE
F	01/31/72	Single	198-26-8878	(917) 231-5873			
SEX (M/F)	DATE OF BIRTH	MARITAL STATUS	SOC. SEC. #	EMPLOYER OR SCHOOL PHONE NUMBER			
			Self	Katrina Johnson, MD			
HOME PHONE		RELATIONSHIP TO GUARANTOR		REFERRED BY			

GUARANTOR INFORMATION

Jermone	Pamela	R.	F	01/31/72	Single	198-26-8878
RESPONSIBLE PARTY LAST NAME	FIRST NAME	MI	SEX (M/F)	DATE OF BIRTH	MARITAL STATUS	SOC. SEC. #
P.O. Box 5673	49 Honey Avenue			Health Lab Corp.		
MAILING ADDRESS	STREET ADDRESS (IF DIFFERENT)			EMPLOYER NAME		
Madison	CA	95653		5 Escada Road		
CITY	STATE	ZIP CODE		EMPLOYER ADDRESS		
(917) 923-4561	(917) 231-5873			Madison	CA	95653
(AREA CODE) HOME PHONE	(AREA CODE) WORK PHONE			CITY	STATE	ZIP CODE

PRIMARY INSURANCE

Pan American Health Ins.			Same		
NAME OF PRIMARY INSURANCE COMPANY			ADDRESS (IF DIFFERENT)		
4567 Newberry Road			Same		
ADDRESS			CITY	STATE	ZIP CODE
Los Angeles	CA	98706	(213) 456-7654		198-26-8878
CITY	STATE	ZIP CODE	PRIMARY INSURANCE PHONE NUMBER		SOC. SEC. #
P970035		HL4578	Self		
IDENTIFICATION #		GROUP NAME AND/OR #	WHAT IS THE RESPONSIBLE PARTY'S RELATIONSHIP TO THE INSURED?		
Pamela Jermone					
INSURED PERSON'S NAME (IF DIFFERENT FROM THE RESPONSIBLE PARTY)					

SECONDARY INSURANCE

NAME OF SECONDARY INSURANCE COMPANY			ADDRESS (IF DIFFERENT)		
ADDRESS			CITY	STATE	ZIP CODE
CITY	STATE	ZIP CODE	SECONDARY INSURANCE PHONE NUMBER		SOC. SEC. #
IDENTIFICATION #		GROUP NAME AND/OR #	WHAT IS THE RESPONSIBLE PARTY'S RELATIONSHIP TO THE INSURED?		
INSURED PERSON'S NAME (IF DIFFERENT FROM THE RESPONSIBLE PARTY)					

I hereby consent for Sydney Carrington & Associates, P.A. to use or disclose my health information to carry out treatment, payment, and health care operations. I authorize the use of this signature on all insurance submissions. I understand that I am financially responsible for all charges whether or not paid by the insurance. I acknowledge receipt of the practice's privacy policy.

Pamela R. Jermone   06/02/2008
PATIENT SIGNATURE   DATE

Figure 10-2 Patient Registration – Gerald Gilmore

Patient Registration Form

Sydney Carrington & Associates
34 Sycamore Street ● Madison, CA 95653

TODAY'S DATE: _06/02/2008_

FOR OFFICE USE ONLY	
ACCOUNT NO.:	338
DOCTOR:	#2
BILL TYPE:	11
EXTENDED INFO.:	2

PATIENT INFORMATION

Gilmore | Gerald
PATIENT LAST NAME | FIRST NAME | MI | SUFFIX

AutoWorks
EMPLOYER OR SCHOOL NAME
13 Bellaire Avenue | Sacramento | CA | 94056
EMPLOYER OR SCHOOL ADDRESS | CITY | STATE | ZIP CODE

MAILING ADDRESS | CITY | STATE | ZIP CODE
M | 04/07/53 | Married | 132-54-7713
SEX (M/F) | DATE OF BIRTH | MARITAL STATUS | SOC. SEC. #

(906) 271-9003
EMPLOYER OR SCHOOL PHONE NUMBER

Self
HOME PHONE | RELATIONSHIP TO GUARANTOR

Richard Bardsley, MD
REFERRED BY

GUARANTOR INFORMATION

Gilmore | Gerald | M
RESPONSIBLE PARTY LAST NAME | FIRST NAME | MI | SEX (M/F)
89 Galley Rd.
MAILING ADDRESS | STREET ADDRESS (IF DIFFERENT)
Sacramento | CA | 94056
CITY | STATE | ZIP CODE
(906) 334-2065 | (906) 271-9003
(AREA CODE) HOME PHONE | (AREA CODE) WORK PHONE

04/07/53 | Married | 132-54-7713
DATE OF BIRTH | MARITAL STATUS | SOC. SEC. #
AutoWorks
EMPLOYER NAME
13 Bellaire Avenue
EMPLOYER ADDRESS
Sacramento | CA | 94056
CITY | STATE | ZIP CODE

PRIMARY INSURANCE

Pan American Health Ins.
NAME OF PRIMARY INSURANCE COMPANY
4567 Newberry Road
ADDRESS
Los Angeles | CA | 98706
CITY | STATE | ZIP CODE
AW1567 | AutoWorks
IDENTIFICATION # | GROUP NAME AND/OR #
Gerald Gilmore
INSURED PERSON'S NAME (IF DIFFERENT FROM THE RESPONSIBLE PARTY)

Same
ADDRESS (IF DIFFERENT)
Same
CITY | STATE | ZIP CODE
(213) 456-7654 | 132-54-7713
PRIMARY INSURANCE PHONE NUMBER | SOC. SEC. #
Self
WHAT IS THE RESPONSIBLE PARTY'S RELATIONSHIP TO THE INSURED?

SECONDARY INSURANCE

NAME OF SECONDARY INSURANCE COMPANY
ADDRESS
CITY | STATE | ZIP CODE
IDENTIFICATION # | GROUP NAME AND/OR #
INSURED PERSON'S NAME (IF DIFFERENT FROM THE RESPONSIBLE PARTY)
ADDRESS (IF DIFFERENT)
CITY | STATE | ZIP CODE
SECONDARY INSURANCE PHONE NUMBER | SOC. SEC. #
WHAT IS THE RESPONSIBLE PARTY'S RELATIONSHIP TO THE INSURED?

I hereby consent for Sydney Carrington & Associates, P.A. to use or disclose my health information to carry out treatment, payment, and health care operations. I authorize the use of this signature on all insurance submissions. I understand that I am financially responsible for all charges whether or not paid by the insurance. I acknowledge receipt of the practice's privacy policy.

Gerald Gilmore | 06/02/2008
PATIENT SIGNATURE | DATE

Figure 10-3 Patient Registration – Joseph Stewart

Patient Registration Form

Sydney Carrington & Associates
34 Sycamore Street • Madison, CA 95653

TODAY'S DATE: ___06/02/2008___

PATIENT INFORMATION

Stewart	Joseph	M		NP Penske, Inc.			
PATIENT LAST NAME	FIRST NAME	MI	SUFFIX	EMPLOYER OR SCHOOL NAME			
				173 Marland Court	Floral City	CA	94064
MAILING ADDRESS	CITY	STATE	ZIP CODE	EMPLOYER OR SCHOOL ADDRESS	CITY	STATE	ZIP CODE
M	01/19/68	Married	144-36-7861	(917) 381-5467			
SEX (M/F)	DATE OF BIRTH	MARITAL STATUS	SOC. SEC. #	EMPLOYER OR SCHOOL PHONE NUMBER			
			Self	Jason Detrasnik, MD			
HOME PHONE		RELATIONSHIP TO GUARANTOR		REFERRED BY			

GUARANTOR INFORMATION

Stewart	Joseph	M	M	01/19/68	Married	144-36-7861
RESPONSIBLE PARTY LAST NAME	FIRST NAME	MI	SEX (M/F)	DATE OF BIRTH	MARITAL STATUS	SOC. SEC. #
600 Pyramid Avenue – Apt. 847				NP Penske, Inc.		
MAILING ADDRESS		STREET ADDRESS (IF DIFFERENT)		EMPLOYER NAME		
Woodside	CA	98076		173 Marland Court		
CITY	STATE	ZIP CODE		EMPLOYER ADDRESS		
(906) 795-2542	(917) 381-5467			Floral City	CA	94064
(AREA CODE) HOME PHONE	(AREA CODE) WORK PHONE			CITY	STATE	ZIP CODE

PRIMARY INSURANCE

Pan American Health Ins.			Same		
NAME OF PRIMARY INSURANCE COMPANY			ADDRESS (IF DIFFERENT)		
4567 Newberry Road			Same		
ADDRESS			CITY	STATE	ZIP CODE
Los Angeles	CA	98706	(213) 456-7654		144-36-7861
CITY	STATE	ZIP CODE	PRIMARY INSURANCE PHONE NUMBER		SOC. SEC. #
86135271			Self		
IDENTIFICATION #	GROUP NAME AND/OR #		WHAT IS THE RESPONSIBLE PARTY'S RELATIONSHIP TO THE INSURED?		
Joseph Stewart					
INSURED PERSON'S NAME (IF DIFFERENT FROM THE RESPONSIBLE PARTY)					

SECONDARY INSURANCE

NAME OF SECONDARY INSURANCE COMPANY			ADDRESS (IF DIFFERENT)		
ADDRESS			CITY	STATE	ZIP CODE
CITY	STATE	ZIP CODE	SECONDARY INSURANCE PHONE NUMBER		SOC. SEC. #
IDENTIFICATION #	GROUP NAME AND/OR #		WHAT IS THE RESPONSIBLE PARTY'S RELATIONSHIP TO THE INSURED?		
INSURED PERSON'S NAME (IF DIFFERENT FROM THE RESPONSIBLE PARTY)					

I hereby consent for Sydney Carrington & Associates, P.A. to use or disclose my health information to carry out treatment, payment, and health care operations. I authorize the use of this signature on all insurance submissions. I understand that I am financially responsible for all charges whether or not paid by the insurance. I acknowledge receipt of the practice's privacy policy.

Joseph Stewart   06/02/2008
PATIENT SIGNATURE   DATE

Figure 10-4 Patient Registration – Steven Sega

Patient Registration Form

Sydney Carrington & Associates
34 Sycamore Street ● Madison, CA 95653

TODAY'S DATE: _06/02/2008_

<table>
<tr><td colspan="2">**FOR OFFICE USE ONLY**</td></tr>
<tr><td>ACCOUNT NO.:</td><td>**340**</td></tr>
<tr><td>DOCTOR:</td><td>**#1**</td></tr>
<tr><td>BILL TYPE:</td><td>**11**</td></tr>
<tr><td>EXTENDED INFO.:</td><td></td></tr>
</table>

PATIENT INFORMATION

Sega	*Steven*	*T*		*Home Front Realty*		
PATIENT LAST NAME	FIRST NAME	MI	SUFFIX	EMPLOYER OR SCHOOL NAME		
				544 Beach Comb Lane	*Woodside*	*CA* | *98076*
MAILING ADDRESS	CITY	STATE	ZIP CODE	EMPLOYER OR SCHOOL ADDRESS	CITY	STATE ZIP CODE
M	*12/02/55*	*Married*	*013-25-7614*	*(917) 287-1445*		
SEX (M/F)	DATE OF BIRTH	MARITAL STATUS	SOC. SEC. #	EMPLOYER OR SCHOOL PHONE NUMBER		
			Self	*James Johnson, MD*		
HOME PHONE		RELATIONSHIP TO GUARANTOR		REFERRED BY		

GUARANTOR INFORMATION

Sega	*Steven*	*T* | *M*	*12/02/55*	*Married*	*013-25-7614*
RESPONSIBLE PARTY LAST NAME	FIRST NAME	MI SEX (M/F)	DATE OF BIRTH	MARITAL STATUS	SOC. SEC. #
2536 Franklin Street			*Home Front Realty*		
MAILING ADDRESS	STREET ADDRESS (IF DIFFERENT)		EMPLOYER NAME		
Floral City	*CA* | *94064*		*544 Beach Comb Lane*		
CITY	STATE ZIP CODE		EMPLOYER ADDRESS		
(906) 796-3125	*(917) 287-1445*		*Woodside*	*CA* |	*98076*
(AREA CODE) HOME PHONE	(AREA CODE) WORK PHONE		CITY	STATE	ZIP CODE

PRIMARY INSURANCE

Pan American Health Ins.		*Same*		
NAME OF PRIMARY INSURANCE COMPANY		ADDRESS (IF DIFFERENT)		
4567 Newberry Road		*Same*		
ADDRESS		CITY	STATE	ZIP CODE
Los Angeles	*CA* | *98706*	*(213) 456-7654*	|	*141-11-3150*
CITY	STATE ZIP CODE	PRIMARY INSURANCE PHONE NUMBER		SOC. SEC. #
BR059116		*Husband*		
IDENTIFICATION #	GROUP NAME AND/OR #	WHAT IS THE RESPONSIBLE PARTY'S RELATIONSHIP TO THE INSURED?		
Rachel Sega				
INSURED PERSON'S NAME (IF DIFFERENT FROM THE RESPONSIBLE PARTY)				

SECONDARY INSURANCE

Epsilon Life and Casualty		*Same*		
NAME OF SECONDARY INSURANCE COMPANY		ADDRESS (IF DIFFERENT)		
P.O. Box 189		*Same*		
ADDRESS		CITY	STATE	ZIP CODE
Macon	*GA* | *31298*	*(800) 908-7654*	|	*013-25-7614*
CITY	STATE ZIP CODE	SECONDARY INSURANCE PHONE NUMBER		SOC. SEC. #
013257614		*Self*		
IDENTIFICATION #	GROUP NAME AND/OR #	WHAT IS THE RESPONSIBLE PARTY'S RELATIONSHIP TO THE INSURED?		
Steven Sega				
INSURED PERSON'S NAME (IF DIFFERENT FROM THE RESPONSIBLE PARTY)				

I hereby consent for Sydney Carrington & Associates, P.A. to use or disclose my health information to carry out treatment, payment, and health care operations. I authorize the use of this signature on all insurance submissions. I understand that I am financially responsible for all charges whether or not paid by the insurance. I acknowledge receipt of the practice's privacy policy.

Steven Sega   *06/02/2008*
PATIENT SIGNATURE   DATE

Figure 10-5   Patient Registration – Linda Century

FOR OFFICE USE ONLY	
ACCOUNT NO.:	**341**
DOCTOR:	**#2**
BILL TYPE:	**11**
EXTENDED INFO.:	**2**

Patient Registration Form

Sydney Carrington & Associates
34 Sycamore Street ● **Madison, CA 95653**

TODAY'S DATE: _06/02/2008_

PATIENT INFORMATION

Century	*Linda*			*Bell Sound, Corp.*
PATIENT LAST NAME	FIRST NAME	MI	SUFFIX	EMPLOYER OR SCHOOL NAME

				8 Kranton Street	*Los Angeles*	*CA* | *98706*
MAILING ADDRESS		CITY	STATE ZIP CODE	EMPLOYER OR SCHOOL ADDRESS	CITY	STATE ZIP CODE

F	*02/27/63*	*Married*	*136-45-2536*	*(916) 474-2536*
SEX (M/F)	DATE OF BIRTH	MARITAL STATUS	SOC. SEC. #	EMPLOYER OR SCHOOL PHONE NUMBER

		Self	*Guy Shelton, MD*
HOME PHONE		RELATIONSHIP TO GUARANTOR	REFERRED BY

GUARANTOR INFORMATION

Century	*Linda*		*F*	*02/27/63*	*Married*	*136-45-2536*
RESPONSIBLE PARTY LAST NAME	FIRST NAME	MI	SEX (M/F)	DATE OF BIRTH	MARITAL STATUS	SOC. SEC. #

14 Candle Lane   *Bell Sound, Corp.*

MAILING ADDRESS	STREET ADDRESS (IF DIFFERENT)	EMPLOYER NAME

Los Angeles	*CA* | *98706*	*8 Kranton Street*
CITY	STATE ZIP CODE	EMPLOYER ADDRESS

(916) 724-6114	*(916) 474-2536*	*Los Angeles*	*CA* | *98706*
(AREA CODE) HOME PHONE	(AREA CODE) WORK PHONE	CITY	STATE ZIP CODE

PRIMARY INSURANCE

Pan American Health Ins.	*Same*
NAME OF PRIMARY INSURANCE COMPANY	ADDRESS (IF DIFFERENT)

4567 Newberry Road	*Same*
ADDRESS	CITY STATE ZIP CODE

Los Angeles	*CA* | *98706*	*(213) 456-7654*	*471-66-2317*
CITY	STATE ZIP CODE	PRIMARY INSURANCE PHONE NUMBER	SOC. SEC. #

429773		*Wife*
IDENTIFICATION #	GROUP NAME AND/OR #	WHAT IS THE RESPONSIBLE PARTY'S RELATIONSHIP TO THE INSURED?

Robert Century
INSURED PERSON'S NAME (IF DIFFERENT FROM THE RESPONSIBLE PARTY)

SECONDARY INSURANCE

NAME OF SECONDARY INSURANCE COMPANY	ADDRESS (IF DIFFERENT)
ADDRESS	CITY STATE ZIP CODE
CITY STATE ZIP CODE	SECONDARY INSURANCE PHONE NUMBER SOC. SEC. #
IDENTIFICATION # GROUP NAME AND/OR #	WHAT IS THE RESPONSIBLE PARTY'S RELATIONSHIP TO THE INSURED?
INSURED PERSON'S NAME (IF DIFFERENT FROM THE RESPONSIBLE PARTY)	

I hereby consent for Sydney Carrington & Associates, P.A. to use or disclose my health information to carry out treatment, payment, and health care operations. I authorize the use of this signature on all insurance submissions. I understand that I am financially responsible for all charges whether or not paid by the insurance. I acknowledge receipt of the practice's privacy policy.

Linda Century	*06/02/2008*
PATIENT SIGNATURE	DATE

EXERCISE 2: POST PROCEDURES AND COPAYMENTS FROM THE PROCEDURE ENTRY SCREEN AND SCHEDULE FOLLOW-UP APPOINTMENTS

1. Use Figures 10-6 through 10-10 to post procedures to patient accounts. Be sure to look at the Amount Paid portion of the encounter forms to determine the copayment paid. Continue to the Appointment screen and schedule the follow-up appointment.

Figure 10-6   Encounter Form – Gerald Gilmore

Sydney Carrington & Associates P.A.
34 Sycamore Street Suite 300
Madison, CA 95653

Date: 06/02/2008   Voucher No.: 1031

Time:

Patient: Gerald Gilmore   Patient No: 338.0
Guarantor: Doctor: 2 – F. Simpson

CPT	DESCRIPTION	FEE
OFFICE/HOSPITAL CONSULTS		
99201	Office New:Focused Hx-Exam	
99202	Office New:Expanded Hx.Exam	
☒ 99211	Office Estb:Min./None Hx-Exa	$25
99212	Office Estb:Focused Hx-Exam	
99213	Office Estb:Expanded Hx-Exa	
99214	Office Estb:Detailed Hx-Exa	
99215	Office Estb:Comprhn Hx-Exam	
99221	Hosp. Initial:Comprh Hx-	
99223	Hosp. Ini:Comprh Hx-Exam/Hi	
99231	Hosp. Subsequent: S-Fwd	
99232	Hosp. Subsequent: Comprhn Hx	
99233	Hosp. Subsequent: Ex/Hi	
99238	Hospital Visit Discharge Ex	
99371	Telephone Consult - Simple	
99372	Telephone Consult - Intermed	
99373	Telephone Consult - Complex	
90840	Counseling - 25 minutes	
90806	Counseling - 50 minutes	
90865	Counseling - Special Interview	
IMMUNIZATIONS/INJECTIONS		
90585	BCG Vaccine	
90659	Influenza Virus Vaccine	
90701	Immunization-DTP	
90702	DT Vaccine	
90703	Tetanus Toxoids	
90732	Pneumococcal Vaccine	
90746	Hepatitis B Vaccine	
90749	Immunization: Unlisted	

CPT	DESCRIPTION	FEE
LABORATORY/RADIOLOGY		
81000	Urinalysis	
81002	Urinalysis; Pregnancy Test	
82951	Glucose Tolerance Test	
84478	Triglycerides	
84550	Uric Acid: Blood Chemistry	
84830	Ovulation Test	
85014	Hematocrit	
85032	Hemogram, Complete Blood Wk	
86403	Particle Agglutination Test	
86485	Skin Test; Candida	
86580	TB Intradermal Test	
86585	TB Tine Test	
87070	Culture	
70190	X-Ray; Optic Foramina	
70210	X-Ray Sinuses Complete	
71010	Radiological Exam Ent Spine	
☒ 71020	X-Ray Chest Pa & Lat	$58
72050	X-Ray Spine, Cerv (4 views)	
72090	X-Ray Spine; Scoliosis Ex	
72110	Spine, lumbosacral; a/p & Lat	
73030	Shoulder-Comp, min w/ 2vws	
73070	Elbow, anteropost & later vws	
73120	X-Ray; Hand, 2 views	
73560	X-Ray; Knee, 1 or 2 views	
74022	X-Ray; Abdomen, Complete	
75552	Cardiac Magnetic Res Img	
76020	X-Ray; Bone Age Studies	
77054	Mammary Ductogram Complete	
78465	Myocardial Perfusion Img	

CPT	DESCRIPTION	FEE
PROCEDURES/TESTS		
00452	Anesthesia for Rad Surgery	
11100	Skin Biopsy	
15852	Dressing Change	
29075	Cast Appl. - Lower Arm	
29530	Strapping of Knee	
29705	Removal/Revis of Cast w/Exa	
53670	Catheterization Incl. Suppl	
57452	Colposcopy	
57505	ECC	
69420	Myringotomy	
92081	Visual Field Examination	
92100	Serial Tonometry Exam	
92120	Tonography	
92552	Pure Tone Audiometry	
92567	Tympanometry	
☒ 93000	Electrocardiogram	$57
93015	Exercise Stress Test (ETT)	
93017	ETT Tracing Only	
93040	Electrocardiogram - Rhythm	
96100	Psychological Testing	
99000	Specimen Handling	
99058	Office Emergency Care	
99070	Surgical Tray - Misc.	
99080	Special Reports of Med Rec	
99195	Phlebotomy	

ICD-9 CODE DIAGNOSIS	
009.0	Infect. colitis, enteritis, & gastroenteritis
133.0	Scabies
174.9	Breast Cancer, Female, Unspecified
185	Malignant neoplasm of prostate
250.00	Diabetes Mellitus w/o mention of Complication
272.4	Hyperlipidemia
282.5	Anemia, Sickle-cell Trait
282.60	Sickle-cell disease, unspecified
285.9	Anemia, Unspecified
300.4	Dysthymic disorder
340	Multiple Sclerosis
342.90	Hemiplegia - Unspec.
346.90	Migraine, unspecified
352.9	Unspecified disorder of cranial nerves
354.0	Carpal Tunnel Syndrome
355.0	Sciatic Nerve Root Lesion
366.9	Cataract
386.00	Menier's disease, unspecified
401.1	Essential Hypertension, Benign
414.9	Ischemic Heart Disease
428.0	Congestive Heart Failure (CHF), unspecified

ICD-9 CODE DIAGNOSIS	
435.0	Basilar Artery Syndrome
440.0	Atherosclerosis
442.81	Carotid Artery
460	Common Cold (Acute Nasopharyngitis)
461.9	Acute Sinusitis
474.00	Chronic Tonsillitis & Adenoiditis
477.9	Allergic Rhinitis, Cause Unspecified
496	Chronic Airway Obstruction
522.0	Pulpitis
524.60	Temporo-Mandibular Joint Disorder - Unspec.
536.8	Stomach Pain
553.3	Hiatal Hernia
564.0	Spastic Colon
574.40	Chronic Hepatitis, Unspecified
571.5	Cirrhosis of Liver w/o mention of alcohol
573.3	Hepatitis
575.2	Obstruction of Gallbladder
☒ 487.0	Influenza with pneumonia
648.20	Anemia - Compl. Pregnancy
715.90	Osteoarthritis - Unspec.
721.3	Lumbar Osteo/Spondylarthrit

ICD-9 CODE DIAGNOSIS	
724.2	Pain: Lower Back
727.67	Rupture of Achilles Tendon
780.1	Hallucinations
780.3	Convulsions, Other
780.50	Sleep Disturbances, Unspecified
783.0	Anorexia
783.1	Abnormal Weight Gain
783.21	Abnormal Weight Loss
823.80	Fractured Tibia
823.81	Fractured Fibula
831.00	Dislocated Shoulder, Closed, Unspecified
835.00	Dislocated Hip, Closed, Unspecified
842.00	Sprained Wrist, Unspecified Site
845.00	Sprained Ankle, Unspecified Site
919.5	Insect Bite, Nonvenomous
921.1	Contus Eyelid/Perioc Area
v16.3	Fam. Hist of Breast Cancer
v17.4	Fam. Hist of Cardiovasc Dis
v20.2	Well Child
v22.0	Pregnancy - First Normal
v22.1	Pregnancy - Normal

Previous Balance	Today's Charges	Total Due	Amount Paid	New Balance
			$10 check #623	

I hereby authorize release of any information acquired in the course of examination or treatment and allow a photocopy of my signature to be used.

Follow Up

PRN _____ Weeks _____ Months _____ Units _____

Next Appointment Date: June 16   Time: 1:15   Follow-up Recheck

Figure 10-7 Encounter Form – Steven Sega

Sydney Carrington & Associates P.A.
34 Sycamore Street Suite 300
Madison, CA 95653

Date: 06/02/2008   Voucher No.: 1032

Time:

Patient: Steven Sega   Patient No: 340.0
Guarantor: Doctor: 1 – J. Monroe

□ CPT	DESCRIPTION	FEE	□ CPT	DESCRIPTION	FEE	□ CPT	DESCRIPTION	FEE
OFFICE/HOSPITAL CONSULTS			**LABORATORY/RADIOLOGY**			**PROCEDURES/TESTS**		
□ 99201	Office New:Focused Hx-Exam		□ 81000	Urinalysis		□ 00452	Anesthesia for Rad Surgery	
□ 99202	Office New:Expanded Hx.Exam		□ 81002	Urinalysis; Pregnancy Test		□ 11100	Skin Biopsy	
□ 99211	Offlce Estb:Min./None Hx-Exa		□ 82951	Glucose Tolerance Test		□ 15852	Dressing Change	
□ 99212	Office Estb:Focused Hx-Exam		□ 84478	Triglycerides		□ 29075	Cast Appl. - Lower Arm	
□ 99213	Office Estb:Expanded Hx-Exa		□ 84550	Uric Acid: Blood Chemistry		□ 29530	Strapping of Knee	
☒ 99214	Office Estb:Detailed Hx-Exa	$50	□ 84830	Ovulation Test		□ 29705	Removal/Revis of Cast w/Exa	
□ 99215	Office Estb:Comprhn Hx-Exam		□ 85014	Hematocrit		□ 53670	Catheterization Incl. Suppl	
□ 99221	Hosp. Initial:Comprh Hx-		□ 85032	Hemogram, Complete Blood Wk		□ 57452	Colposcopy	
□ 99223	Hosp. Ini:Comprh Hx-Exam/Hi		□ 86403	Particle Agglutination Test		□ 57505	ECC	
□ 99231	Hosp. Subsequent: S-Fwd		□ 86485	Skin Test; Candida		□ 69420	Myringotomy	
□ 99232	Hosp. Subsequent: Comprhn Hx		□ 86580	TB Intradermal Test		□ 92081	Visual Field Examination	
□ 99233	Hosp. Subsequent: Ex/Hi		□ 86585	TB Tine Test		□ 92100	Serial Tonometry Exam	
□ 99238	Hospital Visit Discharge Ex		□ 87070	Culture		□ 92120	Tonography	
□ 99371	Telephone Consult - Simple		□ 70190	X-Ray; Optic Foramina		□ 92552	Pure Tone Audiometry	
□ 99372	Telephone Consult - Intermed		□ 70210	X-Ray Sinuses Complete		□ 92567	Tympanometry	
□ 99373	Telephone Consult - Complex		□ 71010	Radiological Exam Ent Spine		□ 93000	Electrocardiogram	
□ 90840	Counseling - 25 minutes		□ 71020	X-Ray Chest Pa & Lat		□ 93015	Exercise Stress Test (ETT)	
□ 90806	Counseling - 50 minutes		□ 72050	X-Ray Spine, Cerv (4 views)		□ 93017	ETT Tracing Only	
□ 90865	Counseling - Special Interview		□ 72090	X-Ray Spine; Scoliosis Ex		□ 93040	Electrocardiogram - Rhythm	
			□ 72110	Spine, lumbosacral; a/p & Lat		□ 96100	Psychological Testing	
IMMUNIZATIONS/INJECTIONS			□ 73030	Shoulder-Comp, min w/ 2vws		□ 99000	Specimen Handling	
□ 90585	BCG Vaccine		□ 73070	Elbow, anteropost & later vws		□ 99058	Office Emergency Care	
□ 90659	Influenza Virus Vaccine		□ 73120	X-Ray; Hand, 2 views		□ 99070	Surgical Tray - Misc.	
□ 90701	Immunization-DTP		□ 73560	X-Ray; Knee, 1 or 2 views		□ 99080	Special Reports of Med Rec	
□ 90702	DT Vaccine		□ 74022	X-Ray; Abdomen, Complete		□ 99195	Phlebotomy	
□ 90703	Tetanus Toxoids		□ 75552	Cardiac Magnetic Res Img		□		
□ 90732	Pneumococcal Vaccine		□ 76020	X-Ray; Bone Age Studies		□		
□ 90746	Hepatitis B Vaccine		□ 77054	Mammary Ductogram Complete		□		
□ 90749	Immunization: Unlisted		□ 78465	Myocardial Perfusion Img		□		

□	**ICD-9 CODE DIAGNOSIS**	□	**ICD-9 CODE DIAGNOSIS**	□	**ICD-9 CODE DIAGNOSIS**
□ 009.0	Infect. colitis, enteritis, & gastroenteritis	□ 435.0	Basilar Artery Syndrome	□ 724.2	Pain: Lower Back
□ 133.0	Scabies	□ 440.0	Atherosclerosis	□ 727.67	Rupture of Achilles Tendon
□ 174.9	Breast Cancer, Female, Unspecified	□ 442.81	Carotid Artery	□ 780.1	Hallucinations
□ 185	Malignant neoplasm of prostate	□ 460	Common Cold (Acute Nasopharyngitis)	□ 780.3	Convulsions, Other
□ 250.00	Diabetes Mellitus w/o mention of Complication	□ 461.9	Acute Sinusitis	□ 780.50	Sleep Disturbances, Unspecified
□ 272.4	Hyperlipidemia	□ 474.00	Chronic Tonsillitis & Adenoiditis	□ 783.0	Anorexia
□ 282.5	Anemia, Sickle-cell Trait	□ 477.9	Allergic Rhinitis, Cause Unspecified	□ 783.1	Abnormal Weight Gain
□ 282.60	Sickle-cell disease, unspecified	□ 487.0	Influenza with pneumonia	□ 783.21	Abnormal Weight Loss
□ 285.9	Anemia, Unspecified	□ 496	Chronic Airway Obstruction	□ 823.80	Fractured Tibia
□ 300.4	Dysthymic disorder	□ 522.0	Pulpitis	□ 823.81	Fractured Fibula
□ 340	Multiple Sclerosis	□ 524.60	Temporo-Mandibular Joint Disorder - Unspec.	□ 831.00	Dislocated Shoulder, Closed, Unspecified
□ 342.90	Hemiplegia - Unspec.	□ 536.8	Stomach Pain	□ 835.00	Dislocated Hip, Closed, Unspecified
□ 346.90	Migraine, unspecified	□ 553.3	Hiatal Hernia	□ 842.00	Sprained Wrist, Unspecified Site
□ 352.9	Unspecified disorder of cranial nerves	☒ 564.1	Spastic Colon	□ 845.00	Sprained Ankle, Unspecified Site
□ 354.0	Carpal Tunnel Syndrome	□ 574.40	Chronic Hepatitis, Unspecified	□ 919.5	Insect Bite, Nonvenomous
□ 355.0	Sciatic Nerve Root Lesion	□ 571.5	Cirrhosis of Liver w/o mention of alcohol	□ 921.1	Contus Eyelid/Perioc Area
□ 366.9	Cataract	□ 573.3	Hepatitis	□ v16.3	Fam. Hist of Breast Cancer
□ 386.00	Menier's disease, unspecified	□ 575.2	Obstruction of Gallbladder	□ v17.4	Fam. Hist of Cardiovasc Dis
□ 401.1	Essential Hypertension, Benign	□ 648.20	Anemia - Compl. Pregnancy	□ v20.2	Well Child
□ 414.9	Ischemic Heart Disease	□ 715.90	Osteoarthritis - Unspec.	□ v22.0	Pregnancy - First Normal
□ 428.0	Congestive Heart Failure (CHF), unspecified	□ 721.3	Lumbar Osteo/Spondylarthrit	□ v22.1	Pregnancy - Normal

Previous Balance	Today's Charges	Total Due	Amount Paid	New Balance
_____			$15 check #112	

Follow Up

PRN _____ Weeks _____ Months _____ Units _____

Next Appointment Date: June 6   Time: 4:00 Personal consult
                                                  30 minutes

I hereby authorize release of any information acquired in the course of
examination or treatment and allow a photocopy of my signature to be used.

_____

Figure 10-8 Encounter Form – Linda Century

Sydney Carrington & Associates P.A.
34 Sycamore Street Suite 300
Madison, CA 95653

Date: 06/02/2008

Time:

Patient: Linda Century
Guarantor:

Voucher No.: 1033

Patient No: 341.0
Doctor: 2 – F. Simpson

□	CPT	DESCRIPTION	FEE
		OFFICE/HOSPITAL CONSULTS	
□	99201	Office New:Focused Hx-Exam	
□	99202	Office New:Expanded Hx.Exam	
□	99211	Office Estb:Min./None Hx-Exa	
□	99212	Office Estb:Focused Hx-Exam	
☒	99213	Office Estb:Expanded Hx-Exa	$40
□	99214	Office Estb:Detailed Hx-Exa	
□	99215	Office Estb:Comprhn Hx-Exam	
□	99221	Hosp. Initial:Comprh Hx-	
□	99223	Hosp. Ini:Comprh Hx-Exam/Hi	
□	99231	Hosp. Subsequent: S-Fwd	
□	99232	Hosp. Subsequent: Comprhn Hx	
□	99233	Hosp. Subsequent: Ex/Hi	
□	99238	Hospital Visit Discharge Ex	
□	99371	Telephone Consult - Simple	
□	99372	Telephone Consult - Intermed	
□	99373	Telephone Consult - Complex	
□	90840	Counseling - 25 minutes	
□	90806	Counseling - 50 minutes	
□	90865	Counseling - Special Interview	
		IMMUNIZATIONS/INJECTIONS	
□	90585	BCG Vaccine	
□	90659	Influenza Virus Vaccine	
□	90701	Immunization-DTP	
□	90702	DT Vaccine	
□	90703	Tetanus Toxoids	
□	90732	Pneumococcal Vaccine	
□	90746	Hepatitis B Vaccine	
□	90749	Immunization: Unlisted	

□	CPT	DESCRIPTION	FEE
		LABORATORY/RADIOLOGY	
☒	81000	Urinalysis	$8
□	81002	Urinalysis; Pregnancy Test	
□	82951	Glucose Tolerance Test	
□	84478	Triglycerides	
□	84550	Uric Acid: Blood Chemistry	
□	84830	Ovulation Test	
☒	85014	Hematocrit	$18
□	85032	Hemogram, Complete Blood Wk	
□	86403	Particle Agglutination Test ·	
□	86485	Skin Test; Candida	
□	86580	TB Intradermal Test	
□	86585	TB Tine Test	
□	87070	Culture	
□	70190	X-Ray; Optic Foramina	
□	70210	X-Ray Sinuses Complete	
□	71010	Radiological Exam Ent Spine	
□	71020	X-Ray Chest Pa & Lat	
□	72050	X-Ray Spine, Cerv (4 views)	
□	72090	X-Ray Spine; Scoliosis Ex	
□	72110	Spine, lumbosacral; a/p & Lat	
□	73030	Shoulder-Comp, min w/ 2vws	
□	73070	Elbow, anteropost & later vws	
□	73120	X-Ray; Hand, 2 views	
□	73560	X-Ray, Knee, 1 or 2 views	
□	74022	X-Ray; Abdomen, Complete	
□	75552	Cardiac Magnetic Res Img	
□	76020	X-Ray; Bone Age Studies	
□	77054	Mammary Ductogram Complete	
□	78465	Myocardial Perfusion Img	

□	CPT	DESCRIPTION	FEE
		PROCEDURES/TESTS	
□	00452	Anesthesia for Rad Surgery	
□	11100	Skin Biopsy	
□	15852	Dressing Change	
□	29075	Cast Appl. - Lower Arm	
□	29530	Strapping of Knee	
□	29705	Removal/Revis of Cast w/Exa	
□	53670	Catheterization Incl. Suppl	
□	57452	Colposcopy	
□	57505	ECC	
□	69420	Myringotomy	
□	92081	Visual Field Examination	
□	92100	Serial Tonometry Exam	
□	92120	Tonography	
□	92552	Pure Tone Audiometry	
□	92567	Tympanometry	
□	93000	Electrocardiogram	
□	93015	Exercise Stress Test (ETT)	
□	93017	ETT Tracing Only	
□	93040	Electrocardiogram - Rhythm	
□	96100	Psychological Testing	
□	99000	Specimen Handling	
□	99058	Office Emergency Care	
□	99070	Surgical Tray - Misc.	
□	99080	Special Reports of Med Rec	
□	99195	Phlebotomy	
□			
□			
□			
□			

□	ICD-9 CODE	DIAGNOSIS
□	009.0	Infect. colitis, enteritis, & gastroenteritis
□	133.0	Scabies
□	174.9	Breast Cancer, Female, Unspecified
□	185	Malignant neoplasm of prostate
□	250.00	Diabetes Mellitus w/o mention of Complication
□	272.4	Hyperlipidemia
□	282.5	Anemia, Sickle-cell Trait
□	282.60	Sickle-cell disease, unspecified
□	285.9	Anemia, Unspecified
□	300.4	Dysthymic disorder
□	340	Multiple Sclerosis
□	342.90	Hemiplegia - Unspec.
□	346.90	Migraine, unspecified
□	352.9	Unspecified disorder of cranial nerves
□	354.0	Carpal Tunnel Syndrome
□	355.0	Sciatic Nerve Root Lesion
□	366.9	Cataract
□	386.00	Menier's disease, unspecified
□	401.1	Essential Hypertension, Benign
□	414.9	Ischemic Heart Disease
□	428.0	Congestive Heart Failure (CHF), unspecified

□	ICD-9 CODE	DIAGNOSIS
□	435.0	Basilar Artery Syndrome
□	440.0	Atherosclerosis
□	442.81	Carotid Artery
□	460	Common Cold (Acute Nasopharyngitis)
□	461.9	Acute Sinusitis
□	474.00	Chronic Tonsillitis & Adenoiditis
□	477.9	Allergic Rhinitis, Cause Unspecified
□	487.0	Influenza with pneumonia
□	496	Chronic Airway Obstruction
□	522.0	Pulpitis
□	524.60	Temporo-Mandibular Joint Disorder - Unspec.
□	536.8	Stomach Pain
□	553.3	Hiatal Hernia
□	564.1	Spastic Colon
□	574.40	Chronic Hepatitis, Unspecified
□	571.5	Cirrhosis of Liver w/o mention of alcohol
□	573.3	Hepatitis
□	575.2	Obstruction of Gallbladder
□	648.20	Anemia - Compl. Pregnancy
□	715.90	Osteoarthritis - Unspec.
□	721.3	Lumbar Osteo/Spondylarthrit

□	ICD-9 CODE	DIAGNOSIS
□	724.2	Pain: Lower Back
□	727.67	Rupture of Achilles Tendon
□	780.1	Hallucinations
□	780.3	Convulsions, Other
□	780.50	Sleep Disturbances, Unspecified
☒	783.0	Anorexia
□	783.1	Abnormal Weight Gain
□	783.21	Abnormal Weight Loss
□	823.80	Fractured Tibia
□	823.81	Fractured Fibula
□	831.00	Dislocated Shoulder, Closed, Unspecified
□	835.00	Dislocated Hip, Closed, Unspecified
□	842.00	Sprained Wrist, Unspecified Site
□	845.00	Sprained Ankle, Unspecified Site
□	919.5	Insect Bite, Nonvenomous
□	921.1	Contus Eyelid/Perioc Area
□	v16.3	Fam. Hist of Breast Cancer
□	v17.4	Fam. Hist of Cardiovasc Dis
□	v20.2	Well Child
□	v22.0	Pregnancy - First Normal
□	v22.1	Pregnancy - Normal

Previous Balance	Today's Charges	Total Due	Amount Paid	New Balance
			$10 check #1029	

Follow Up

PRN _____ Weeks _____ Months _____ Units _____

Next Appointment Date: July 1   Time: 10:30 General Check-up 30 minutes

I hereby authorize release of any information acquired in the course of examination or treatment and allow a photocopy of my signature to be used.

_____

Figure 10-9   Encounter Form – Pamela Jermone

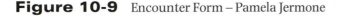

Sydney Carrington & Associates P.A.
34 Sycamore Street Suite 300
Madison, CA 95653

Date: 06/02/2008   Voucher No.: 1034

Time:

Patient: Pamela Jermone   Patient No: 337.0
Guarantor: Doctor: 1 – J. Monroe

☐ CPT	DESCRIPTION	FEE	☐ CPT	DESCRIPTION	FEE	☐ CPT	DESCRIPTION	FEE
OFFICE/HOSPITAL CONSULTS			**LABORATORY/RADIOLOGY**			**PROCEDURES/TESTS**		
☐ 99201	Office New:Focused Hx-Exam	___	☒ 81000	Urinalysis	$8	☐ 00452	Anesthesia for Rad Surgery	___
☐ 99202	Office New:Expanded Hx.Exam	___	☐ 81002	Urinalysis; Pregnancy Test	___	☐ 11100	Skin Biopsy	___
☐ 99211	Offlce Estb:Min./None Hx-Exa	___	☐ 82951	Glucose Tolerance Test	___	☐ 15852	Dressing Change	___
☐ 99212	Office Estb:Focused Hx-Exam	___	☐ 84478	Triglycerides	___	☐ 29075	Cast Appl. - Lower Arm	___
☐ 99213	Office Estb:Expanded Hx-Exa	___	☐ 84550	Uric Acid: Blood Chemistry	___	☐ 29530	Strapping of Knee	___
☒ 99214	Office Estb:Detailed Hx-Exa	$50	☐ 84830	Ovulation Test	___	☐ 29705	Removal/Revis of Cast w/Exa	___
☐ 99215	Office Estb:Comprhn Hx-Exam	___	☐ 85014	Hematocrit	___	☐ 53670	Catheterization Incl. Suppl	___
☐ 99221	Hosp. Initial:Comprh Hx-	___	☐ 85032	Hemogram, Complete Blood Wk	___	☐ 57452	Colposcopy	___
☐ 99223	Hosp. Ini:Comprh Hx-Exam/Hi	___	☐ 86403	Particle Agglutination Test	___	☐ 57505	ECC	___
☐ 99231	Hosp. Subsequent: S-Fwd	___	☐ 86485	Skin Test; Candida	___	☐ 69420	Myringotomy	___
☐ 99232	Hosp. Subsequent: Comprhn Hx	___	☐ 86580	TB Intradermal Test	___	☐ 92081	Visual Field Examination	___
☐ 99233	Hosp. Subsequent: Ex/Hi	___	☐ 86585	TB Tine Test	___	☐ 92100	Serial Tonometry Exam	___
☐ 99238	Hospital Visit Discharge Ex	___	☐ 87070	Culture	___	☐ 92120	Tonography	___
☐ 99371	Telephone Consult - Simple	___	☐ 70190	X-Ray; Optic Foramina	___	☐ 92552	Pure Tone Audiometry	___
☐ 99372	Telephone Consult - Intermed	___	☐ 70210	X-Ray Sinuses Complete	___	☐ 92567	Tympanometry	___
☐ 99373	Telephone Consult - Complex	___	☐ 71010	Radiological Exam Ent Spine	___	☒ 93000	Electrocardiogram	$57
☐ 90840	Counseling - 25 minutes	___	☐ 71020	X-Ray Chest Pa & Lat	___	☐ 93015	Exercise Stress Test (ETT)	___
☐ 90806	Counseling - 50 minutes	___	☐ 72050	X-Ray Spine, Cerv (4 views)	___	☐ 93017	ETT Tracing Only	___
☐ 90865	Counseling - Special Interview	___	☐ 72090	X-Ray Spine; Scoliosis Ex	___	☐ 93040	Electrocardiogram - Rhythm	___
			☐ 72110	Spine, lumbosacral; a/p & Lat	___	☐ 96100	Psychological Testing	___
IMMUNIZATIONS/INJECTIONS			☐ 73030	Shoulder-Comp, min w/ 2vws	___	☐ 99000	Specimen Handling	___
☐ 90585	BCG Vaccine	___	☐ 73070	Elbow, anteropost & later vws	___	☐ 99058	Office Emergency Care	___
☐ 90659	Influenza Virus Vaccine	___	☐ 73120	X-Ray; Hand, 2 views	___	☐ 99070	Surgical Tray - Misc.	___
☐ 90701	Immunization-DTP	___	☐ 73560	X-Ray, Knee, 1 or 2 views	___	☐ 99080	Special Reports of Med Rec	___
☐ 90702	DT Vaccine	___	☐ 74022	X-Ray; Abdomen, Complete	___	☐ 99195	Phlebotomy	___
☐ 90703	Tetanus Toxoids	___	☐ 75552	Cardiac Magnetic Res Img	___	☐	___	___
☐ 90732	Pneumococcal Vaccine	___	☐ 76020	X-Ray; Bone Age Studies	___	☐	___	___
☐ 90746	Hepatitis B Vaccine	___	☐ 77054	Mammary Ductogram Complete	___	☐	___	___
☐ 90749	Immunization: Unlisted	___	☐ 78465	Myocardial Perfusion Img	___	☐	___	___

☐	ICD-9 CODE DIAGNOSIS		☐	ICD-9 CODE DIAGNOSIS		☐	ICD-9 CODE DIAGNOSIS
☐ 009.0	Infect. colitis, enteritis, & gastroenteritis		☐ 435.0	Basilar Artery Syndrome		☐ 724.2	Pain: Lower Back
☐ 133.0	Scabies		☐ 440.0	Atherosclerosis		☐ 727.67	Rupture of Achilles Tendon
☐ 174.9	Breast Cancer, Female, Unspecified		☐ 442.81	Carotid Artery		☐ 780.1	Hallucinations
☐ 185	Malignant neoplasm of prostate		☐ 460	Common Cold (Acute Nasopharyngitis)		☐ 780.3	Convulsions, Other
☐ 250.00	Diabetes Mellitus w/o mention of Complication		☐ 461.9	Acute Sinusitis		☐ 780.50	Sleep Disturbances, Unspecified
☐ 272.4	Hyperlipidemia		☐ 474.00	Chronic Tonsillitis & Adenoiditis		☐ 783.0	Anorexia
☐ 282.5	Anemia, Sickle-cell Trait		☐ 477.9	Allergic Rhinitis, Cause Unspecified		☐ 783.1	Abnormal Weight Gain
☐ 282.60	Sickle-cell disease, unspecified		☐ 487.0	Influenza with pneumonia		☐ 783.21	Abnormal Weight Loss
☐ 285.9	Anemia, Unspecified		☐ 496	Chronic Airway Obstruction		☐ 823.80	Fractured Tibia
☐ 300.4	Dysthymic disorder		☐ 522.0	Pulpitis		☐ 823.81	Fractured Fibula
☐ 340	Multiple Sclerosis		☐ 524.60	Temporo-Mandibular Joint Disorder - Unspec.		☐ 831.00	Dislocated Shoulder, Closed, Unspecified
☐ 342.90	Hemiplegia - Unspec.		☐ 536.8	Stomach Pain		☐ 835.00	Dislocated Hip, Closed, Unspecified
☐ 346.90	Migraine, unspecified		☐ 553.3	Hiatal Hernia		☐ 842.00	Sprained Wrist, Unspecified Site
☐ 352.9	Unspecified disorder of cranial nerves		☐ 564.1	Spastic Colon		☐ 845.00	Sprained Ankle, Unspecified Site
☐ 354.0	Carpal Tunnel Syndrome		☐ 574.40	Chronic Hepatitis, Unspecified		☐ 919.5	Insect Bite, Nonvenomous
☐ 355.0	Sclatic Nerve Root Lesion		☐ 571.5	Cirrhosis of Liver w/o mention of alcohol		☐ 921.1	Contus Eyelid/Perioc Area
☐ 366.9	Cataract		☐ 573.3	Hepatitis		☐ v16.3	Fam. Hist of Breast Cancer
☐ 386.00	Menier's disease, unspecified		☐ 575.2	Obstruction of Gallbladder		☐ v17.4	Fam. Hist of Cardiovasc Dis
☐ 401.1	Essential Hypertension, Benign		☐ 648.20	Anemia - Compl. Pregnancy		☐ v20.2	Well Child
☐ 414.9	Ischemic Heart Disease		☐ 715.90	Osteoarthritis - Unspec.		☐ v22.0	Pregnancy - First Normal
☐ 428.0	Congestive Heart Failure (CHF), unspecified		☐ 721.3	Lumbar Osteo/Spondylarthrit		☐ v22.1	Pregnancy - Normal
						X 480.0	Viral Pneumonia

Previous Balance	Today's Charges	Total Due	Amount Paid	New Balance
___	___	___	$5 check #103	___

Follow Up

PRN _____ Weeks _____   Months _____ Units _____

Next Appointment Date: June 17   Time: 9:15 Recheck

I hereby authorize release of any information acquired in the course of
examination or treatment and allow a photocopy of my signature to be used.

_____

Figure 10-10 Encounter Form – Joseph Stewart

Sydney Carrington & Associates P.A.
34 Sycamore Street Suite 300
Madison, CA 95653

Date: 06/02/2008

Time:

Patient: Joseph Stewart
Guarantor:

Voucher No.: 1035

Patient No: 339.0

Doctor: 3 – S. Carrington

	CPT	DESCRIPTION	FEE
OFFICE/HOSPITAL CONSULTS			
☐	99201	Office New:Focused Hx-Exam	
☐	99202	Office New:Expanded Hx.Exam	
☐	99211	Office Estb:Min./None Hx-Exa	
☐	99212	Office Estb:Focused Hx-Exam	
☒	99213	Office Estb:Expanded Hx-Exa	$40
☐	99214	Office Estb:Detailed Hx-Exa	
☐	99215	Office Estb:Comprhn Hx-Exam	
☐	99221	Hosp. Initial:Comprh Hx-	
☐	99223	Hosp. Ini:Comprh Hx-Exam/Hi	
☐	99231	Hosp. Subsequent: S-Fwd	
☐	99232	Hosp. Subsequent: Comprhn Hx	
☐	99233	Hosp. Subsequent: Ex/Hi	
☐	99238	Hospital Visit Discharge Ex	
☐	99371	Telephone Consult - Simple	
☐	99372	Telephone Consult - Intermed	
☐	99373	Telephone Consult - Complex	
☐	90840	Counseling - 25 minutes	
☐	90806	Counseling - 50 minutes	
☐	90865	Counseling - Special Interview	
IMMUNIZATIONS/INJECTIONS			
☐	90585	BCG Vaccine	
☐	90659	Influenza Virus Vaccine	
☐	90701	Immunization-DTP	
☐	90702	DT Vaccine	
☐	90703	Tetanus Toxoids	
☐	90732	Pneumococcal Vaccine	
☐	90746	Hepatitis B Vaccine	
☐	90749	Immunization: Unlisted	

	CPT	DESCRIPTION	FEE
LABORATORY/RADIOLOGY			
☒	81000	Urinalysis	$8
☐	81002	Urinalysis; Pregnancy Test	
☐	82951	Glucose Tolerance Test	
☐	84478	Triglycerides	
☐	84550	Uric Acid: Blood Chemistry	
☐	84830	Ovulation Test	
☐	85014	Hematocrit	
☐	85032	Hemogram, Complete Blood Wk	
☐	86403	Particle Agglutination Test	
☐	86485	Skin Test; Candida	
☐	86580	TB Intradermal Test	
☐	86585	TB Tine Test	
☐	87070	Culture	
☐	70190	X-Ray; Optic Foramina	
☐	70210	X-Ray Sinuses Complete	
☐	71010	Radiological Exam Ent Spine	
☐	71020	X-Ray Chest Pa & Lat	
☐	72050	X-Ray Spine, Cerv (4 views)	
☐	72090	X-Ray Spine; Scoliosis Ex	
☐	72110	Spine, lumbosacral; a/p & Lat	
☐	73030	Shoulder-Comp, min w/ 2vws	
☐	73070	Elbow, anteropost & later vws	
☐	73120	X-Ray; Hand, 2 views	
☐	73560	X-Ray, Knee, 1 or 2 views	
☐	74022	X-Ray; Abdomen, Complete	
☐	75552	Cardiac Magnetic Res Img	
☐	76020	X-Ray; Bone Age Studies	
☐	77054	Mammary Ductogram Complete	
☐	78465	Myocardial Perfusion Img	

	CPT	DESCRIPTION	FEE
PROCEDURES/TESTS			
☐	00452	Anesthesia for Rad Surgery	
☐	11100	Skin Biopsy	
☐	15852	Dressing Change	
☐	29075	Cast Appl. - Lower Arm	
☐	29530	Strapping of Knee	
☐	29705	Removal/Revis of Cast w/Exa	
☐	53670	Catheterization Incl. Suppl	
☐	57452	Colposcopy	
☐	57505	ECC	
☐	69420	Myringotomy	
☐	92081	Visual Field Examination	
☐	92100	Serial Tonometry Exam	
☐	92120	Tonography	
☐	92552	Pure Tone Audiometry	
☐	92567	Tympanometry	
☐	93000	Electrocardiogram	
☐	93015	Exercise Stress Test (ETT)	
☐	93017	ETT Tracing Only	
☐	93040	Electrocardiogram - Rhythm	
☐	96100	Psychological Testing	
☐	99000	Specimen Handling	
☐	99058	Office Emergency Care	
☐	99070	Surgical Tray - Misc.	
☐	99080	Special Reports of Med Rec	
☐	99195	Phlebotomy	
☐		_____	
☐		_____	
☐		_____	

	ICD-9 CODE DIAGNOSIS
☐ 009.0	Infect. colitis, enteritis, & gastroenteritis
☐ 133.0	Scabies
☐ 174.9	Breast Cancer, Female, Unspecified
☐ 185	Malignant neoplasm of prostate
☐ 250.00	Diabetes Mellitus w/o mention of Complication
☐ 272.4	Hyperlipidemia
☐ 282.5	Anemia, Sickle-cell Trait
☐ 282.60	Sickle-cell disease, unspecified
☐ 285.9	Anemia, Unspecified
☐ 300.4	Dysthymic disorder
☐ 340	Multiple Sclerosis
☐ 342.90	Hemiplegia - Unspec.
☐ 346.90	Migraine, unspecified
☐ 352.9	Unspecified disorder of cranial nerves
☐ 354.0	Carpal Tunnel Syndrome
☐ 355.0	Sciatic Nerve Root Lesion
☐ 366.9	Cataract
☐ 386.00	Menier's disease, unspecified
☐ 401.1	Essential Hypertension, Benign
☐ 414.9	Ischemic Heart Disease
☐ 428.0	Congestive Heart Failure (CHF), unspecified

	ICD-9 CODE DIAGNOSIS
☐ 435.0	Basilar Artery Syndrome
☐ 440.0	Atherosclerosis
☐ 442.81	Carotid Artery
☐ 460	Common Cold (Acute Nasopharyngitis)
☐ 461.9	Acute Sinusitis
☐ 474.00	Chronic Tonsillitis & Adenoiditis
☐ 477.9	Allergic Rhinitis, Cause Unspecified
☐ 487.0	Influenza with pneumonia
☐ 496	Chronic Airway Obstruction
☐ 522.0	Pulpitis
☐ 524.60	Temporo-Mandibular Joint Disorder - Unspec.
☐ 536.8	Stomach Pain
☐ 553.3	Hiatal Hernia
☐ 564.1	Spastic Colon
☐ 574.40	Chronic Hepatitis, Unspecified
☐ 571.5	Cirrhosis of Liver w/o mention of alcohol
☐ 573.3	Hepatitis
☐ 575.2	Obstruction of Gallbladder
☐ 648.20	Anemia - Compl. Pregnancy
☐ 715.90	Osteoarthritis - Unspec.
☐ 721.3	Lumbar Osteo/Spondylarthrit

	ICD-9 CODE DIAGNOSIS
☒ 724.2	Pain: Lower Back
☐ 727.67	Rupture of Achilles Tendon
☐ 780.1	Hallucinations
☐ 780.3	Convulsions, Other
☐ 780.50	Sleep Disturbances, Unspecified
☐ 783.0	Anorexia
☐ 783.1	Abnormal Weight Gain
☐ 783.21	Abnormal Weight Loss
☐ 823.80	Fractured Tibia
☐ 823.81	Fractured Fibula
☐ 831.00	Dislocated Shoulder, Closed, Unspecified
☐ 835.00	Dislocated Hip, Closed, Unspecified
☐ 842.00	Sprained Wrist, Unspecified Site
☐ 845.00	Sprained Ankle, Unspecified Site
☐ 919.5	Insect Bite, Nonvenomous
☐ 921.1	Contus Eyelid/Perioc Area
☐ v16.3	Fam. Hist of Breast Cancer
☐ v17.4	Fam. Hist of Cardiovasc Dis
☐ v20.2	Well Child
☐ v22.0	Pregnancy - First Normal
☐ v22.1	Pregnancy - Normal

Previous Balance	Today's Charges	Total Due	Amount Paid	New Balance
_____	_____	_____	$5 check #2003	

Follow Up

PRN _____ Weeks _____   Months _____ Units _____

Next Appointment Date: June 3   Time: 1:30 X-ray

I hereby authorize release of any information acquired in the course of
examination or treatment and allow a photocopy of my signature to be used.

EXERCISE 3: ADD A DEPENDENT TO AN EXISTING ACCOUNT

1. Use Figure 10-11 to enter a dependent to Gerald Gilmore's account.

Figure 10-11   Patient Registration – Sondra Gilmore

Patient Registration Form

Sydney Carrington & Associates
34 Sycamore Street ● Madison, CA 95653

TODAY'S DATE: _06/02/2008_

FOR OFFICE USE ONLY	
ACCOUNT NO.:	338
DOCTOR:	#2
BILL TYPE:	11
EXTENDED INFO.:	0

PATIENT INFORMATION

Gilmore	Sondra			
PATIENT LAST NAME	FIRST NAME	MI	SUFFIX	EMPLOYER OR SCHOOL NAME

MAILING ADDRESS	CITY	STATE	ZIP CODE	EMPLOYER OR SCHOOL ADDRESS CITY STATE ZIP CODE

F	06/23/54	Married	017-31-5416	
SEX (M/F)	DATE OF BIRTH	MARITAL STATUS	SOC. SEC. #	EMPLOYER OR SCHOOL PHONE NUMBER

	Wife	Richard Bardsley, MD
HOME PHONE	RELATIONSHIP TO GUARANTOR	REFERRED BY

GUARANTOR INFORMATION

Gilmore	Gerald	M	04/07/53	Married	132-54-7113
RESPONSIBLE PARTY LAST NAME	FIRST NAME	MI SEX (M/F)	DATE OF BIRTH	MARITAL STATUS	SOC. SEC. #

89 Galley Road		AutoWorks
MAILING ADDRESS	STREET ADDRESS (IF DIFFERENT)	EMPLOYER NAME

Sacramento	CA	94056	13 Bellaire Avenue
CITY	STATE	ZIP CODE	EMPLOYER ADDRESS

(906) 334-2065	(906) 271-9003	Sacramento	CA	94056
(AREA CODE) HOME PHONE	(AREA CODE) WORK PHONE	CITY	STATE	ZIP CODE

PRIMARY INSURANCE

Pan American Health Ins.	Same
NAME OF PRIMARY INSURANCE COMPANY	ADDRESS (IF DIFFERENT)

4567 Newberry Road	Same
ADDRESS	CITY STATE ZIP CODE

Los Angeles	CA	98706	(213) 456-7654	132-54-7113
CITY	STATE	ZIP CODE	PRIMARY INSURANCE PHONE NUMBER	SOC. SEC. #

AW1567	AutoWorks	Self
IDENTIFICATION #	GROUP NAME AND/OR #	WHAT IS THE RESPONSIBLE PARTY'S RELATIONSHIP TO THE INSURED?

Gerald Gilmore
INSURED PERSON'S NAME (IF DIFFERENT FROM THE RESPONSIBLE PARTY)

SECONDARY INSURANCE

NAME OF SECONDARY INSURANCE COMPANY	ADDRESS (IF DIFFERENT)

ADDRESS	CITY STATE ZIP CODE

CITY	STATE	ZIP CODE	SECONDARY INSURANCE PHONE NUMBER SOC. SEC. #

IDENTIFICATION #	GROUP NAME AND/OR # WHAT IS THE RESPONSIBLE PARTY'S RELATIONSHIP TO THE INSURED?

INSURED PERSON'S NAME (IF DIFFERENT FROM THE RESPONSIBLE PARTY)

I hereby consent for Sydney Carrington & Associates, P.A. to use or disclose my health information to carry out treatment, payment, and health care operations. I authorize the use of this signature on all insurance submissions. I understand that I am financially responsible for all charges whether or not paid by the insurance. I acknowledge receipt of the practice's privacy policy.

Sondra Gilmore	06/02/2008
PATIENT SIGNATURE	DATE

EXERCISE 4: EDIT PATIENT ACCOUNT INFORMATION

1. Based on the information provided, update patient accounts.

   a. Change Joseph Stewart's apartment number to 307 and telephone number to (906) 245-1957.

   b. For Steven Sega's work phone number add a work extension of 3996 to account.

   c. Add the group name 'Bell' to Linda Century's insurance information.

EXERCISE 5: EDIT APPOINTMENTS

1. Based on the information provided, update patient appointments.

   a. Pamela Jermone called to reschedule her recheck appointment for 11:30 on June 18.

   b. Steven Sega called to cancel his appointment.